Pessaries in Clinical Practice

Pessaries in Clinical Practice

Scott A. Farrell (Ed.)

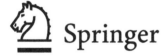 Springer

Scott A. Farrell, BA, BEd, MD, FRCSC
Professor
Department of Obstetrics and Gynaecology
Dalhousie University
Halifax, Nova Scotia
Canada

Cover illustration: Extract from *Pessaries Through the Ages*, by Renee Forrestall.

British Library Cataloguing in Publication Data
Pessaries in clinical practice
  1. Pessaries
  I. Farrell, Scott A.
  618.1′44062
  ISBN-13: 9781846281631
  ISBN-10: 1846281636

Library of Congress Control Number: 2005937769

ISBN-10: 1-84628-163-6   e-ISBN-10: 1-84628-315-9
ISBN-13: 978-1-84628-163-1   e-ISBN-13: 978-1-84628-315-4

Printed on acid-free paper

Dr. Scott A. Farrell is the inventor of the Uresta pessary and principal shareholder
in EastMed Inc., manufacturer of Uresta.

9 8 7 6 5 4 3 2 1

Springer Science+Business Media
springer.com

Preface

The pessary has been a component of the armamentarium for the management of pelvic organ prolapse for more than a millennium.[1] Prior to the modern age of surgery, a pessary represented the only viable option for women with symptomatic pelvic organ prolapse. Modern clinicians tend to view the pessary with a mixture of disdain and reluctance.[2] Training in obstetrics and gynecology programs, at least in North America, typically provides cursory experience with pessary selection and care, and tends to minimize its importance. The modern gynecologic surgeon relies primarily on surgical intervention for the management of pelvic organ prolapse and urinary incontinence,[3] and resorts to the use of pessaries only in cases where surgical intervention is contraindicated by medical problems.

To the pessary novice, pessaries come in a bewildering variety of shapes and sizes with imprecise indications for selection. Guidance will vary depending on the article one reads or the expert one subscribes to. Given that there is a lack of consistent and reliable guidelines for the use of different pessary models, most clinicians tend to become familiar with a few pessary models, which they utilize to the exclusion of most others.[4]

This book proposes a new rationale for the selection of pessaries, both for prolapse and urinary incontinence. The selection, fitting, insertion, and removal of the most commonly used pessaries are described and illustrated in detail. It is the contention of this book that the modern pessary should take a central place in the management of both pelvic organ prolapse and urinary incontinence. Pessaries are in fact much more welcome to women than many healthcare providers believe. The establishment of a healthcare team familiar with pessary care and the implementation of a simplified pessary care protocol makes the work of the healthcare provider easier. Pessaries are effective for the management not only of pelvic organ prolapse but also of urinary incontinence.[5,6] Newer models of incontinence pessaries are highly effective and user-friendly. By providing detailed instructions on the fitting and care of popular pessary models, this book endeavors to convert skeptics to believers in using pessaries as a part of their clinical practice, and to confirm the practice of those who already employ pessaries on a regular basis.

I hope this book facilitates the acquisition of confidence for pessary care novices and provides an aid to refining the practice of those who are already expert in pessary care.

ACKNOWLEDGMENTS

I would like to acknowledge with gratitude my collaborators who have provided invaluable contributions to researching and writing this book. Renee Forrestall's painstaking and creative efforts resulted in the excellent illustrations and the cover design.

References

1. Miller DS. Contemporary use of the pessary. In: Drogemueller W, Sciarra JJ, eds. Gynecology and Obstetrics. Philadelphia: JB Lippincott, 1992:1–12.
2. Novak E. The vaginal pessary: its indications and limitations. JAMA 1923;80:1294–1298.
3. Cundiff GW, Weidner AC, Visco AG, Bump R, Addison WA. A survey of pessary use by members of the American Urogynecologic Society. Obstet Gynecol 2000;95:931–935.
4. Wu V, Farrell SA, Baskett TF, Flowerdew G. A simplified protocol for pessary management. Obstet Gynecol 1997;90:990–994.
5. Farrell SA, Singh B, Aldakhil L. Continence pessaries in the management of urinary incontinence in women. J Obstet Gynaecol Can 2004;26:113–117.
6. Donnelly MJ, Powell-Morgan S, Olsen AL, Nygaard I. Vaginal pessaries for the management of stress and mixed urinary incontinence. Int Urogynecol J 2004;15:302–307.

Scott A. Farrell
Halifax, Nova Scotia, Canada

Contents

Contributors

Baharak Amir-Khalkhali, BSc, MD, Department of Obstetrics and Gynaecology, IWK Health Centre, Dalhousie University, Halifax, Nova Scotia, Canada

Thomas F. Baskett, MB, FRCS, FRCOG, Department of Obstetrics and Gynaecology, Dalhousie University, Halifax, Nova Scotia, Canada

Sandra A. Baydock, BSc, MD, FRCSC, Department of Obstetrics and Gynaecology, University of Alberta, Edmonton, Alberta, Canada

Karen D. Farrell, BA, BSc, MA, School of Health and Human Performance, Dalhousie University, Halifax, Nova Scotia, Canada

Scott A. Farrell, BA, BEd, MD, FRCSC, Department of Obstetrics and Gynaecology, Dalhousie University, Halifax, Nova Scotia, Canada

Joan M. Foren, RN, Urogynaecology Clinic, IWK Health Centre, Halifax, Nova Scotia, Canada

Linda E. Irving, RN, Urogynaecology Clinic, IWK Health Centre, Halifax, Nova Scotia, Canada

Jane E. Twohig, RN, Urogynaecology Clinic, IWK Health Centre, Halifax, Nova Scotia, Canada

Chapter 1

The History of Pessaries for Uterovaginal Prolapse

Thomas F. Baskett

The word *pessary* is derived from the Greek *pessos* and the Latin *pessarium*, meaning an oval-shaped stone. The word *suppository* is derived from the Latin *suppositorium*, meaning to place underneath. Both pessaries and suppositories were used to administer drugs vaginally, but the suppository was generally made of a medicated substance that was solid at room temperature, melted at body temperature, and did not have to be removed.[1] The pessary was a more solid object covered or soaked in the medication, which was removed after the period of time deemed necessary for the medication to act. Historically, pessaries have been used to treat menstrual irregularities, dysmenorrhea, infertility, incompetent cervix, and malposition of the uterus, in addition to uterovaginal prolapse.[2,3]

There is reference to uterine prolapse in both the Kahun papyrus (circa 2000 B.C.) and the Ebers papyrus (circa 1500 B.C.).[1,4] The earliest surviving medical text on obstetrics and gynecology is that of Soranus (A.D. 98–138); his book *On the Diseases of Women* survived many translations, but was thought to be lost until a 15th-century Greek manuscript was rediscovered in the Bibliothèque Royale in Paris in the 19th century.[5,6] Soranus reviewed a number of the techniques used for management of uterovaginal prolapse in the time of Hippocrates. He was critical of Euryphon of Cnidius, a celebrated contemporary of Hippocrates, who advocated succussion. This treatment involved suspending the woman upside down by her feet from a ladder-like frame that was then moved rapidly up and down for a few minutes to reduce the prolapse. The woman remained suspended in this position for up to 1 day (Figure 1.1). He also criticized other physicians of the Hippocratic era who inserted ox meat into the vagina and those who applied "a hairy bag to the uterus, so that the organ may suffer pain from the sharp hair and con-

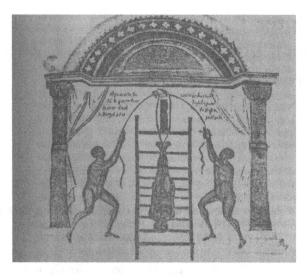

FIGURE 1.1. Succussion for uterovaginal prolapse.

tract. They are not aware that paralyzed parts do not suffer any pain while parts that feel pain contract for a little while and prolapse again."[6] One of the most common treatments he observed was as follows: "The majority administered pleasant aromas to smell, while they apply fumigations to the uterus of an opposite character; and they believe that now the uterus like an animal flees the bad odours and turns towards the good ones."[6] Soranus summarized these treatments from the Hippocratic era but condemned their use as harmful, unpleasant, or ineffective. His own treatment for uterine prolapse was as follows:

One should bathe the prolapsed part of the uterus with much lukewarm olive oil, and make a woolen tampon corresponding in shape and diameter to the vagina and wrap it in very thin clean linen. Afterwards one should dip it briefly in diluted vinegar or the juice of acacia or of hypocist mixed with wine, apply it to the uterus and move the whole prolapsed part, forcing it up gently until the uterus has reverted to its proper place and the whole mass of wool is in the vagina.[6]

The woman's legs were then extended and bandaged together and she remained at rest for 3 days, after which the wool and linen pessary was removed. If the uterus prolapsed again, the treatment was repeated. Diocles of Carystos (350 B.C.) used half of a peeled pomegranate soaked in vinegar as a pessary for uterine prolapse.[6,7] Others would use wool and linen pessaries soaked in astringents to reduce discharge and bleeding, and to cause contraction of the vaginal tissues. Some of the more bizarre approaches included application of a red-hot iron to the cervix to stimulate it to recede into the vagina, and tying mice and lizards (presumably dead) to the prolapsed uterus to frighten it back to the correct position.[8]

Through the Middle Ages, there was little advance in the type and use of pessaries.[9] Ambroise Paré (1510–1590), the innovative French surgeon, devised a number of oval-shaped pessaries for uterine prolapse made of hard brass or of waxed cork.[5,7,10] Hendrick van Deventer[11] (1651–1724) clearly described the use of pessaries, which he produced himself, for uterovaginal prolapse in 1701. He outlined the situation with uterovaginal prolapse thus:

Descent of the womb, in which case the ligaments as well as the fibres of the uterus are too much relaxed, and the bladder is too much drawn down; whence proceeds, as we said above, an incontinency of urine, and a continual descent or falling down of the womb or vagina out of the body, which occasions a great many inconveniencies. . . . A remedy may be found for this malady. . . . Pessaries may be made fit for that purpose, to hinder its falling down, and hold the womb up . . . pessaries, being so useful, that they hinder not copulation with a husband, which virgins may also use, troubled with the falling down of the womb or vagina for other reasons.[11]

Van Deventer, who started his career as a goldsmith, made these pessaries of cork, wood, silver, or gold. Those made with cork or wood were waxed to avoid rotting (Figure 1.2).

Through the 18th and early 19th centuries, a more precise knowledge of the anatomy and function of the pelvic organs developed. Thus, uterine prolapse, cystocele, rectocele, and enterocele were defined more clearly. The 19th century was the golden age of the pessary. Just about any complaint that a woman produced, that could even remotely be connected with the pelvic organs, would potentially fall prey to the use of a pessary to correct "uterine malalignment." Uterine anteversion, retroversion, lateral displacement, or prolapse was considered the cause of many gynecological complaints. Gaillard Thomas, a prominent American gynecologist, presented his views on the evils of uterine anteflexion to the American Gynecological Society in 1888[12]:

As a rule, given a decidedly anteflexed uterus in a menstrual woman, and the result will be an invalid. . . . She will suffer from some of these symptoms: nervous disorders, ovarian disturbances, derangements of

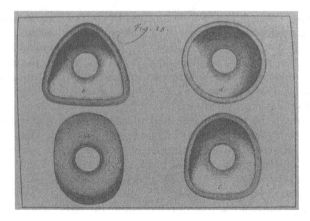

FIGURE 1.2. Hendrick van Deventer's pessaries for uterovaginal prolapse. (From van Deventer.[11])

menstruation, sterility, or tendency to abortion, excessive gastric trouble during utero-gestation, marked tendency to vesical irritation, and troubles of vision.

At the same society's meeting some 7 years later, in 1895, Paul Mundé denounced the use of pessaries for uterine anteversion, saying, "Increasing experience has taught us that symptoms of anteflexion, even of the major degrees, are practically nil."[12] Another American gynecologist, W.D. Buck of New Hampshire, in 1865 decried the excessive manipulation of the uterus: "What with burning and cauterizing, cutting and slashing, and gouging, and spitting, and skewering, and pessarying, the old fashioned womb will cease to exist except in history. . . . Pessaries, I suppose, are sometimes useful, but there are more than there is any necessity for. . . . I do think that this filling of the vagina with traps, making a Chinese toy shop of it, is outrageous."[13] The type of pessary that created the most opposition was the stem pessary, in which the narrow stem portion was placed in the cervix. While this may have been effective in correcting the uterine ante- or retroflexion, it usually caused more pain and infection.[12,14] As Goodell[15] put it, "But the endometrium often resents the intrusion of such a foreign body, and some hazards attend its use."

Some idea of the plethora of pessaries that were available in the late 19th century can be seen from Figure 1.3, taken from William Goodell's[15] 1889 text *Lessons in Gynecology*. The pessaries used most commonly in the clinical management of

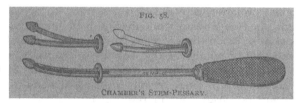

a

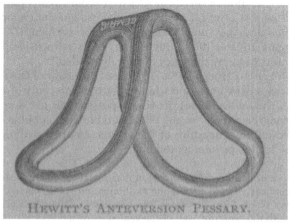

b

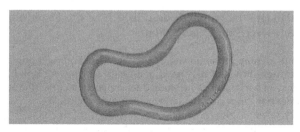

c

FIGURE 1.3. Nineteenth-century intravaginal pessaries. (From Goodell.[15])

uterovaginal prolapse were the ring pessary, with or without diaphragm, the Hodge pessary, and the Smith modification of the Hodge pessary.[5,16–20] In those women in whom intravaginal pessaries could not be retained, either because of extensive vaginal prolapse or a deficient perineum, more elaborate types of pessaries were developed. These usually involved ring-and-stem or cup-and-stem pessaries kept in position by a perineal strap, which was in turn attached to a waist band (Figure 1.4).[15,21] The clinical application of these combined external-vaginal pessaries was limited: "As a set-off, their presence is a constant source of annoyance and they are liable to chafe the perineum. . . . The instruments are so stiff, so unyielding, and so expensive that it is a comfort to know that they are rarely needed."[15]

Hugh Lennox Hodge (1796–1873) was Professor of Obstetrics and Diseases of Women and Children at the University of Pennsylvania. The innovation of the Hodge pessary was to change the shape from the circular to the oblong and to add a double curve that followed the curvature of the vagina. Hodge[12] outlined the rationale for his pessary as follows:

The important modification consists in making a ring oblong instead of circular and curved as to correspond to the curvature of the vagina. Great advantages result from this form; the convexity of the curve being in contact with the posterior wall of the vagina, corresponds with more or less accuracy to the curve of the rectum, perineum and sacrum.

One of Hodge's biographer's described how the inspiration for the double-lever shape came about:

Sitting one evening in the university his eyes rested on the upright steel support designed to hold the shovel and tongs, which were kept in position by a steel hook, and as he studied its supporting curve, the longed-for illumination came and the lever pessary was the result.[5]

Alfred Holmes Smith (1835–1885), also a gynecologist in Philadelphia, modified the Hodge pessary by narrowing the front, subpubic end and widening the posterior limb. This became the Smith–Hodge pessary, which was used for uterine prolapse, although its most common indication was to correct uterine retroversion, to which many gynecological woes were ascribed in the 19th and early 20th century.[5]

With the extensive use of pessaries, one of the more common problems became that of the "forgotten pessary." Howard Kelly[23] (1858–1943) described a case with a ring pessary "made of cloth covered with an impervious paint and stuffed with fibre." This

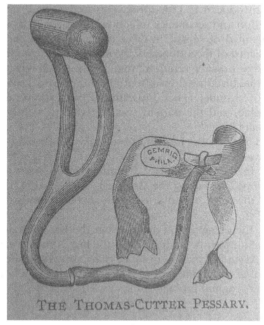

a

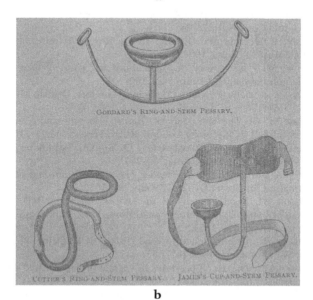

b

FIGURE 1.4. Combined external/vaginal pessaries. (From Goodell.[15])

had been introduced 15 years previously and caused such extensive ulceration and secondary infection that, despite its removal, the woman died of sepsis. In what must be one of the longest cases on record of forgotten pessary, a 90-year-old woman had a Smith–Hodge pessary removed that had been in place for 57 years. Vaginal bleeding drew attention to the pessary, which had to be removed under general anesthesia but without any long-term sequelae, and the patient was reported as being in good health 4 years later.[24]

In 1783, rubber was introduced to make pessaries, and in the 1950s it was replaced by plastic, and most recently by silicone.[16,25,26] In the 20th century a number of different pessaries were developed including the Gellhorn, the Gehrung, the Inflatoball, and the cube, in addition to the most commonly used ring pessary.[10,16,27]

Just as the pessary was overused in the late 19th and early 20th century, it may be underused in the late 20th and early 21st centuries. As an alternative to more risky surgery in the frail or elderly, it offers a simple and safe alternative for relief of symptomatic uterovaginal prolapse.

References

1. McKay WJS. The History of Ancient Gynaecology. London: Balliere, Tindal and Cox, 1901:278–285.
2. Jackson R. Doctors and Diseases in the Roman Empire. London: British Museum Press, 1998:92.
3. O'Dowd MJ. The History of Medications for Women. New York: Parthenon Publishing Group, 2001:100–101.
4. Nunn JF. Ancient Egyptian Medicine. London: British Museum Press, 1996:196.
5. Baskett TF. On The Shoulders of Giants: Eponyms and Names in Obstetrics and Gynaecology. London: RCOG Press, 1996:94, 215, 217.
6. Soranus' Gynaecology. Translated by O. Temkin. Baltimore: Johns Hopkins University Press, 1956:200–207.
7. Emge LA, Durfee RB. Pelvic organ prolapse: four thousand years of treatment. Clin Obstet Gynecol 1966;9:997–1032.
8. Harrison GT. Displacements of the uterus. In: Mann MD, ed. A System of Gynecology by American Authors. Vol 2. Philadelphia: Lea Brothers, 1888:1091–1153.
9. Garrison FH. An Introduction to the History of Medicine. Philadelphia: W.B. Saunders, 1929:167, 603.
10. Vierhout ME. The use of pessaries in vaginal prolapse. Eur J Obstet Gynaecol Reprod Biol 2004;117:4–9.
11. Van Deventer H. The Art of Midwifery Improved. London: E. Curll, 1716:145.

12. Speert H. Obstetrics and Gynecology in America: A History. Chicago: American College of Obstetricians and Gynecologists, 1980:59, 60, 66.
13. Graham H. Eternal Eve: The History of Gynaecology and Obstetrics. New York: Doubleday, 1951:497.
14. Bernutz MG, Goupil ME. Clinical Memoirs on the Diseases of Women, vol 1. London: New Sydenham Society, 1886:231.
15. Goodell W. Lessons in Gynecology. 3rd ed. Philadelphia: P.A. Davis, 1889:155–214.
16. Deger RD, Menzin AW, Mikuta JJ. Vaginal pessary: past and present. Postgrad Obstet Gynecol 1993;13:1–7.
17. Ricci JV. The Development of Gynecological Surgery and Instruments. Philadelphia: Blakiston, 1949.
18. Skene AJC. Treatise on the Diseases of Women. New York: D. Appleton, 1889:334–342.
19. Speert H. Obstetrics and Gynecology: A History and Iconography, 2nd ed. San Francisco: Norman Publishing, 1994:463–471.
20. Speert H. Obstetric and Gynecologic Milestones. New York: Parthenon Publishing Group, 1996:545–551.
21. Bell WB. The Principles of Gynaecology. London: Longmans, Green and Co., 1910:189.
22. Hodge HL. On Diseases Peculiar to Women, Including Displacements of the Uterus. Philadelphia: Blanchard and Lea, 1860.
23. Kelly HA. Operative Gynecology. Vol 1. New York: D. Appleton, 1898:240.
24. Summers JL, Ford ML. The forgotten pessary: a medical oddity. Am J Obstet Gynecol 1971;111:307–308.
25. Anders K. Devices for continence and prolapse. Br J Obstet Gynaecol 2004;111(suppl):61–66.
26. Bash KL. Review of vaginal pessaries. Obstet Gynecol Surv 2000;55:455–460.
27. Sulak PJ, Kuehl TJ, Shull BL. Vaginal pessaries and their use in pelvic relaxation. J Reprod Med 1993;38:919–923.

Chapter 2

Pessaries for Pelvic Organ Prolapse: The Evidence

Sandra A. Baydock

2.1 OUTLINE

Research concerning the indications and effectiveness of pessaries has been scant. This chapter discusses the following issues:

1. Predictors of successful pessary fitting, patient satisfaction, and continued use
2. Evidence supporting the use of specific pessaries for specific pelvic support problems
3. Complications associated with pessary care
4. Pessary follow-up protocols
5. Current pessary practice among health care professionals

2.2 INTRODUCTION

Intravaginal devices for the treatment of pelvic organ prolapse have been used since antiquity.[1] Over the last century, more than 100 articles have been written concerning the use of modern pessaries for prolapse. Unfortunately, most of published pessary studies consist of case reports, case series, or expert opinion, which provides only level III evidence to guide the practice of pessary care. To date, only a handful of prospective and retrospective pessary trials have been reported, and there are no randomized controlled trials on the use of pessaries for prolapse.[2] This chapter focuses on the available evidence concerning pessary use for pelvic organ prolapse, and summarizes the current published recommendations for the selection and use of modern pessaries.

2.3 PREDICTORS OF SUCCESSFUL FITTING

2.3.1 Patient Preference for a Pessary

Patients with pelvic organ prolapse have three treatment options: expectant management, use of a pessary, or surgery. Heit et al[3] examined factors that predicted patients' treatment choices. They found a positive association between increasing age and preference for a pessary over surgery. Women who had undergone previous prolapse surgery and those with more severe prolapse, defined by a more advanced leading edge of the prolapse, were more likely to opt for surgery over a pessary. Heit et al also found that older women and women with more severe prolapse were more likely to choose pessary use over expectant management.

2.3.2 Patient Factors Influencing Fitting Success

Based on the two available prospective studies of pessary fitting, the likelihood of being able to successfully fit a woman with a pessary ranges from 74% to 94%.[4,5] While up to 46% of patients may require a refitting within the first week of use, eventually 73% are successfully fitted.[5] There is very little agreement in the literature regarding factors that predict a successful pessary fitting.[6-11] Some experts suggest poor perineal support or a large posterior defect are risk factors for unsuccessful pessary fitting.[12-14]

Higher stage of prolapse is not predictive of higher pessary fitting failure rates.[4-6] Wu et al,[4] Mutone et al,[6] and Hanson et al[11] all found prior pelvic surgery reduced the likelihood of successful fitting. Wu et al also noted that preexisting stress incontinence was a negative predictor of successful fitting, whereas Clemons et al[5] determined that a vaginal length of less than 6 cm and a wide introitus ($\geq$4 fingerbreadths) were predictive of unsuccessful fitting. Mutone et al noted a higher failure rate for initial pessary fitting among women with a significant posterior vaginal wall support defect.

2.3.3 Patient Satisfaction and Relief of Prolapse Symptoms

Two studies examined patient satisfaction with pessaries.[9,10] Satisfaction rates ranged from 70% to 92%. Pessaries have been shown to reduce or eliminate the common symptoms associated with prolapse. These included a reduction in discomfort associated with prolapsing tissues from 90% to 3%, a decrease in the sensation of pelvic pressure from 49% to 3%, vaginal discharge decrease from 12% to 0%, and reduction in the need to splint to empty the bladder or for defecation from 49% to 3%.[9]

Pelvic organ prolapse is associated with symptoms of both voiding dysfunction and urinary incontinence. The only study that compared symptoms at baseline to those after pessary use demonstrated that over half of women with voiding dysfunction improved with pessary use.[9] Forty-six percent of women with urge urinary incontinence and 45% of women with stress urinary incontinence noted an improvement in their symptoms while using a pessary. Unfortunately, pessaries unmask latent stress incontinence in approximately 22% of patients, which is similar to the rate of de novo stress incontinence after prolapse surgery.[10] Persistent stress incontinence is a significant cause of pessary fitting failure and discontinuation.[4]

Pessaries may also help prevent the progression of prolapse. Handa and Jones[15] studied the effect of pessary use on prolapse stage. Overall, there was a significant improvement from baseline in pelvic organ prolapse quantification (POP-Q) stage after pessary use, even when the pessary had been removed for up to 48 hours. Improvement was most often seen along the anterior vaginal wall, where 33% of patients with anterior wall prolapse had an improvement in POP-Q stage.

2.4 PREDICTORS OF CONTINUED PESSARY USE

The attrition rate among pessary users is highest during the first 12 months.[5] For patients fitted successfully with a pessary, 41% to 73% continue pessary use for at least 1 year.[4,7] Life-table analysis shows that of women who are successfully fitted and satisfied at 1 month, 66% will still be using a pessary at 1 year and 53% at 36 months.[4]

The most common reasons patients give for discontinuation of a pessary included desire for surgery, development or persistence of incontinence, failure of the pessary to adequately support their prolapse, intolerable prolapse symptoms, vaginal discharge, and erosions and pelvic pain.[4,6,8,9]

Two prospective series determined that opting to continue pessary use after 1 to 2 months was predictive of continued use for up to 36 months.[4,7] Older age is also predictive of continued pessary use. In one study an age of ≥65 years was predictive of pessary use for up to 1 year. This same study found that beginning at 40 years of age, pessary use of ≥1 year increased by 10% to 20% per decade of life,[7] supporting the contention that pessaries are an acceptable treatment option in younger patients. Mutone et al[6] found that women fitted with a support type of pessary were more likely to continue using a pessary. Factors shown to be negatively predictive of continued pessary use at 1 year were stage III/IV posterior wall prolapse and an expressed desire for surgery at the first visit.[7] In a retrospective study, more severe prolapse was found to be associated with continued pessary use during an average follow-up period of 16 months.[8]

2.5 APPLICATION OF PESSARY DESIGNS TO SPECIFIC PELVIC SUPPORT DEFECTS

Prevailing expert opinion holds that pessary choice is determined by specific vaginal defects,[1,12,14] despite the fact that no clinical trials support this contention.[4,8,9] While the published pessary trials included a wide variety of pessary types, three types of pessaries were most often used for all types and degrees of defect: the ring, the Gellhorn, and the cube.[4,5,6,11] Clemons et al[5] were able to treat prolapse in any vaginal compartment by using only ring or Gellhorn pessaries. They demonstrated that the ring pessary was used successfully to fit all patients with stage II and the majority of patients with stage III prolapse. Among those with stage IV prolapse, 64% were successfully fitted with a Gellhorn versus 36% successfully fitted with a ring pessary. Wu et al[4] found that the majority of successful fitted patients (96%) were fitted with a ring pessary, and 70% with a ring size 3, 4, or 5. Clemons et al observed that 83% of successfully fitted patients used just six pessaries: the ring sizes 3, 4, and 5, and the Gellhorn sizes 2.5, 2.75, and 3 inches.

2.6 COMPLICATIONS OF PESSARY USE

Several case reports and series have implicated pessaries as the cause of serious complications such as fistulae, vaginal cancer, and evisceration.[16–18] When these reports are reviewed, most of these complications occurred in women with lost or neglected pessaries or in patients where follow-up did not include vaginal examinations.[16,17] Women who developed vaginal and cervical cancer had been using their pessary for an average duration of 18 years.[18] When women receive regular pessary follow-up care, complications are minor and include vaginal discharge, odor, bleeding, abrasions, and erosions. Other problems include a sensation of the pessary slipping or pelvic discomfort from an ill-fitted pessary (either too large or too small) and de novo or persistent stress urinary incontinence.[4,9,10] Wu et al[4] found an association between vaginal mucosal thinness and subsequent vaginal abrasions, but no correlation between abrasions and current hormone replacement therapy. Hanson et al[11] found a higher rate of pessary continuation in women using local vaginal hormone replacement. The potential for either local or systemic estrogen replacement to prevent local vaginal complications from pessary use has not been formally evaluated.

2.7 PESSARY FOLLOW-UP

Wu et al[4] examined a simplified protocol for pessary management. After an initial 2-week follow-up visit, subsequent visits were scheduled at 3-month intervals for the first year and 6-

month intervals for complication-free patients in subsequent years. Each follow-up visit included pessary removal and cleaning with tap water and speculum examination of the vagina. The reported complication rates in this series were low and consisted primarily of vaginal abrasions. Clemons et al[7] described a similar protocol in their series, but women who managed their own pessary were seen every 6 to 12 months, while 2-month follow-up intervals were encouraged for women who relied on their doctor to remove their pessary. These authors found a similarly low rate of complications.

2.8 CURRENT PESSARY USE AMONG HEALTHCARE PROFESSIONALS

A survey of the members of the American Urogynecology Society (AUGS) was conducted to ascertain current pessary practices.[19] The respondents consisted of urogynecologists, obstetrician–gynecologists, gynaecologists, and urologists.

Ninety-eight percent used pessaries in their practices but only 77% offered pessaries as first-line treatment for prolapse. Twelve percent used pessaries only in women unfit for surgery. Those who practiced urology or gynecology alone as well as those in practice for greater than 20 years were less likely to use pessaries. Respondents identified the following contraindications for pessary use: prior hysterectomy (42%), sexual activity (45%), and hypoestrogenism (64%). While there is no evidence to support a policy of using specific pessaries for a specific compartmental defect, 89% of respondents used pessaries for anterior defects, 75% used pessaries for vaginal apical defects, and 60% used pessaries for posterior wall prolapse. Twenty-two percent of respondents used the same type of pessary, primarily the ring pessary, for all defects. Seventy-eight percent tailored the choice of pessary to the defect being treated. Most commonly used pessaries included the ring and Hodge pessaries for anterior and posterior defects, and the Gellhorn, ring, and donut pessary for apical defects. Physicians in this study also believed that a weak pelvic diaphragm (59%) and prior hysterectomy (44%) were indications for choosing a space-filling pessary (donut or Gellhorn) rather than a support pessary, such as a ring. Ninety-four percent of repondents recommend estrogen therapy for pessary users, and 64% stated that they recommend pelvic floor exercises. There was no consensus on follow-up or care instructions given to patients. Fifty-three percent teach all pessary users self-care, but 45% believe this is appropriate only for patients with support pessaries. Ninety-two percent of respondents agreed that pessaries relieve the symptoms of prolapse, but only 48% believe that pessaries have other therapeutic benefits such as decreasing the severity of prolapse.[19]

2.9 SUMMARY AND REVIEW OF KEY POINTS

Research evidence provides some insight into factors that are predictive of pessary fitting success and continued use of a pessary. There is very little scientific evidence to guide pessary selection. Pessary related complications are minimal when an appropriate follow-up care plan is used.

KEY POINTS
1. Older women are more likely to choose treatment of their prolapse with a pessary rather than surgery and to continue using a pessary once successfully fitted.
2. Up to three quarters of patients who opt to try a pessary can be successfully fitted.
3. Factors that negatively affect pessary fitting success include prior vaginal surgery, a short vagina, a wide introitus, and a significant posterior vaginal wall defect.
4. Patient satisfaction with pessaries is generally high, but persistent or new urinary incontinence often prompts pessary discontinuation in favor of surgery.
5. The ring pessary can be used successfully to fit most prolapse cases that do not exceed stage III. Stage IV prolapse is more often successfully treated with a Gellhorn pessary.
6. The most common complications encountered with pessary use include vaginal abrasions (bleeding), discharge, and odor.
7. Pessary follow-up intervals of 2 to 3 months are appropriate for women who rely on a health care professional to remove their pessary. Intervals of 6 to 12 months are appropriate for asymptomatic women who remove their pessary at regular intervals (at least weekly) for cleaning.
8. Current pessary practices vary widely among healthcare professionals.

References
1. Bash KL. Review of vaginal pessaries. Obstet Gynecol Surv 2000; 55(7):455–460.
2. Adams E, Thomson A, Maher C, Hagen S. Mechanical devices for pelvic organ prolapse in women. Cochrane Database of Systematic Reviews 2004, Issue 2, CD004010. DOI: 10.1002/14651858.CD004010.pub2.

3. Heit M, Rosenquist C, Culligan P, Graham C, Murphy M, Shott S. Predicting treatment choice for patients with pelvic organ prolapse. Obstet Gynecol 2003;101(6):1279–1284.
4. Wu V, Farrell SA, Baskett TF, Flowerdew G. A simplified protocol for pessary management. Obstet Gynecol 1997;90:990–994.
5. Clemons JL, Aguilar VC, Tillinghast TA, Jackson ND, Myers DL. Risk factors associated with an unsuccessful pessary fitting trial in women with pelvic organ prolapse. Am J Obstet Gynecol 2004;190:345–350.
6. Mutone MF, Terry C, Hale DS, Bensen JT. Factors which influence the short-term success of pessary management of pelvic organ prolapse. Am J Obstet Gynecol 2005;173:89–94.
7. Clemons JL, Aguilar VC, Sokol ER, Jackson ND, Myers DL. Patient characteristics that are associated with continued pessary use versus surgery after 1 year. Am J Obstet Gynecol 2004;191:159–164.
8. Sulak PJ, Kuehl TJ, Shull BL. Vaginal pessaries and their use in pelvic relaxation. J Reprod Med 1993;38(12):919–923.
9. Clemons JL, Aguilar VC, Tillinghast TA, Jackson ND, Myers DL. Patient satisfaction and changes in prolapse and urinary symptoms in women who were fitted with a pessary for pelvic organ prolapse. Am J Obstet Gynecol 2004;190:1025–1029.
10. Bai SW, Yoon BS, Kwon JY, Shin JS, Kim SK, Park KH. Survey of the characteristics and satisfaction degree of the patients using a pessary. Int Urogynecol J 2006;17(2):155–159.
11. Hanson LM, Schulz JA, Flood GC, Cooley B, Tam F. Vaginal pessaries in managing women with pelvic organ prolapse and urinary incontinence: patient characteristics and factors contributing to success. Int Urogynecol J 2005 (e-published).
12. Viera AJ, Larkins-Pettigrew M. Practical use of the pessary. Am Fam Physician 2000;61(9):2719–2726.
13. Pott-Grinstein E, Newcomer JR. Gynecologists patterns of prescribing pessaries. J Reprod Med 2001;46(3):205–208.
14. Zeitlin MP, Lebherz TB. Pessaries in the geriatric patient. J Am Geriatr Soc 1992;40(6):635–640.
15. Handa VL, Jones M. Do pessaries prevent the progression of pelvic organ prolapse? Int Urogynecol J 2002;13:349–352.
16. Oh R, Richter H, Behr J, Scheeld J. Small bowel prolapse and incarceration caused by a vaginal ring pessary. Br J Surg 1993;80:1157.
17. Russell JK. The dangerous pessary. Br Med J 1961;2:1595–1597.
18. Schraub A, Sun XS, Maingon P, et al. Cervical and vaginal cancer associated with pessary use. Cancer 1992;69(10):2505–2509.
19. Cundiff GW, Weidner AC, Visco AG, Bump RC, Addison WA. A survey of pessary use be members of the American Urogynecology Society. Obstet Gynecol 2000;95(6):931–935.

Chapter 3

Pessaries for the Management of Urinary Incontinence: The Evidence

Baharak Amir-Khalkhali

3.1 OUTLINE

Stress urinary incontinence is a very prevalent condition. It is caused by a failure of the urethral sphincter mechanism. Continence pessaries are designed to correct the problem with the sphincter mechanism by restoring proper support to the urethra. This chapter discusses the following issues:

1. The prevalence of urinary incontinence
2. The causes of stress incontinence
3. The evidence for the effectiveness of continence pessaries
4. Factors that predict successful use of a continence pessary
5. Factors affecting patient satisfaction and continuation of pessary use

3.2 PREVALENCE OF URINARY INCONTINENCE

Urinary incontinence is a common chronic medical condition in women. The prevalence of urinary incontinence among elderly, institutionalized patients has been estimated to be between 40% and 60%.[1] Stress urinary incontinence affects 27% of noninstitutionalized elderly women.[2] Among 45-year-old women, its prevalence is approximately 22%.[3] In a recent large European survey, 35% of respondents reported experiencing incontinence in the previous 30 days. The majority complained of stress incontinence.[4] Stress urinary incontinence is a widespread, expensive problem that generates substantial costs annually.[5,6]

It is not uncommon for patients to wait a significant length of time before seeking help for their urinary incontinence problem. Reluctance to seek treatment may often be due to social isolation and embarrassment, fear of painful investigations or surgical treatment, and a lack of familiarity with conservative measures that could alleviate symptoms. Many patients ignore mild or occasional symptoms until they worsen to the point when they significantly affect quality of life. With such a high prevalence and cost associated with genuine stress urinary incontinence and an aging population, there is a need for an inexpensive, yet effective alternative to surgical treatment.

3.3 PATHOPHYSIOLOGY OF STRESS INCONTINENCE

One of the primary pathophysiologic mechanisms of stress urinary incontinence is the incomplete transmission of intraabdominal pressure to the proximal urethra due to the displacement of the proximal urethra from its normal intraabdominal location (Figure 3.1). Damage to the normal urethral support is caused by vaginal delivery, chronically increased intraabdominal

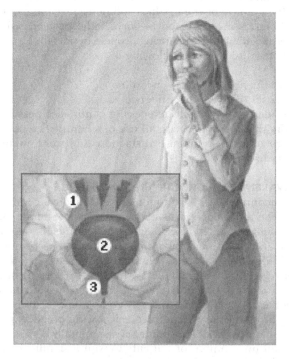

FIGURE 3.1. The intraabdominal pressure (1) caused by a cough, applies pressure to the bladder (2). The urethral (3) must counteract this pressure to prevent leaking.

pressure as with chronic obstructive pulmonary disease (COPD), or repetitive heavy lifting.

There are four major components of the urinary continence mechanism that prevent stress incontinence by working together to maintain urethral pressure and to allow complete pressure transmission[7]:

1. Intrinsic urethral sphincter complex
   a. Urethral mucosa
   b. Smooth muscle fibres
   c. Vascular submucosal plexus
2. Extrinsic urethral sphincter
3. Correct anatomic position of the urethrovesical junction
4. Intact innervation

Most women with genuine stress urinary incontinence have an intact intrinsic urethral sphincter component and intact innervation.[8] The goal of surgical procedures such as the Burch colposuspension and tension-free vaginal tape (TVT) is to restore continence by correcting the deficiency in the external support of the urethrovesical junction. Continence pessaries can be used to achieve the same support without the need for surgery.

3.4 EFFECTIVENESS OF PESSARIES FOR THE MANAGEMENT OF STRESS INCONTINENCE

The mechanism by which the continence pessary is believed to restore continence is similar to that achieved with surgery. The continence pessary stabilizes the urethrovesical junction and allows complete transmission of intraabdominal pressure to the urethra. A pessary may also help by increasing urethral closure pressure. This is particularly true of pessaries designed for incontinence such as the incontinence ring (Milex, Chicago, Illinois, USA), which has a knob that, when positioned correctly, supports the urethra (Figure 3.2).

The medical literature examining the use of vaginal pessaries for the treatment of urinary incontinence has a paucity of information. A Cochrane Library Review Protocol established to examine the effect of mechanical devices on urinary incontinence in women was subsequently withdrawn in 2003 because of a lack of research evidence.[9] This lack of research evidence has been observed for pessaries in general, as Adams et al[10] in 2004 found no evidence from randomized controlled trials on which to base management with mechanical devices in women with pelvic organ prolapse.

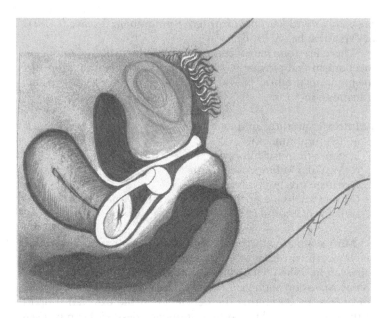

FIGURE 3.2. Proper placement of the incontinence ring pessary. The knob of the incontinence ring stabilizes the urethra to prevent leaking.

Several small studies have examined the effect of vaginal pessaries on symptoms of urinary incontinence.[11-17] Three studies considered the effect of pessaries specifically designed to treat urinary incontinence.[11-13] Donnelly et al[12] and Farrell et al[13] have shown that over 50% of women with pure stress or mixed urinary incontinence who were treated with continence pessaries were satisfied with their results and continued pessary use. Robert and Mainprize[11] had a 24% cure rate. The discrepancy between the results of Robert and Mainprize and those of Donnelly et al and Farrell et al may be explained in part by the fact that Robert and Mainprize used different models of incontinence pessaries and may have used different methodology for pessary fitting. Baydock and Farrell[15] reported in a recent abstract on the effectiveness of a new continence pessary. In a prospective trial of 15 patients, the Uresta (EastMed Inc., Halifax, Nova Scotia, Canada) pessary significantly reduced stress and urge incontinence questionnaire scores and reduced pad weights. Seventy-three percent of subjects continued use of Uresta after the 2-week follow-up visit.

Clemens et al[14] also demonstrated improvement in urinary symptoms in women who were treated for pelvic organ prolapse with standard ring and Gellhorn pessaries. Among women with concurrent urinary symptoms at baseline, stress incontinence improved in 45%, urge incontinence improved in 46%, and voiding difficulties improved in 53% at 2 months. Among women without baseline urinary difficulties, 21% developed de novo stress and 6% de novo urge incontinence following treatment with pessaries.

3.5 PREDICTORS OF SUCCESSFUL CONTINENCE PESSARY FITTING

Three published studies have examined factors affecting the success of continence pessary fitting.[11-13] All three studies included women with both stress and mixed incontinence symptoms. The mean ages of the study populations ranged from 50 to 56 years. Robert and Mainprize[11] systematically excluded women with detrusor instability proven by urodynamics testing.

These three published studies examined several risk factors for continence pessary failure:

1. *Age*. Farrell et al[13] found there was no effect of age. Robert and Mainprize[11] noted a trend toward higher success rates in younger women.
2. *Previous pelvic surgery*. Donnelly et al[12] found previous pelvic surgery or hysterectomy reduced success rates. Farrell et al found previous incontinence surgery reduced success rates.
3. *Pelvic prolapse*. Donnelly et al found no effect of genital prolapse >3 cm. Robert and Mainprize and Farrell et al found no significant difference in grades of prolapse between those who successfully used a pessary and those who did not.
4. *Type of incontinence pessary*. Farrell et al found no difference in success rates between the incontinence ring and the ring with support and knob.
5. *Incontinence symptoms*. Farrell et al found no effect of incontinence symptoms (pure stress vs. mixed incontinence) on success rates.

3.6 PATIENT SATISFACTION AND RELIEF OF INCONTINENCE

Success rates varied considerably among studies.[11-14] While Robert and Mainprize[11] had a very high persistent incontinence rate (69%) and a success rate of only 24% at 1 year, Donnelly et al[12] found a success rate of 55% at 6 months and Farrell et al[13] a 59% success rate at 11 months. All authors defined success as an improvement in a patient's subjective symptoms and her desire to continue to use the pessary.

3.7 COMPLICATIONS AND REASONS FOR DISCONTINUATION OF A CONTINENCE PESSARY

Reasons for pessary discontinuation included persistent incontinence (18–69%), discomfort (10–33%), pessary expulsion (10–18%), and difficulty with defecation (3–5%). Complications associated with continence pessary use were minor and included vaginal discharge and bleeding. The most frequent option chosen by women who stopped using a continence pessary was surgery (20–41%).[12,13]

3.8 SUMMARY AND REVIEW OF KEY POINTS

Patients with urinary incontinence have three distinct goals[18]:

1. They want an explanation for their urinary symptoms.
2. They want an effective therapy.
3. They want to minimize the inconvenience and discomfort of investigations and treatments.

At present, there are only four options for the management of stress urinary incontinence: absorbent pads, Kegel's exercises, incontinence pessaries, and surgery. Studies have found that the long-term efficacy of both Kegel's exercises and surgery is 28%.[19,20] While Kegel's exercises do not involve risk or complications, surgery involves significant risk. The 55% to 59% efficacy of continence pessaries compares very favorably to the 28% efficacy of surgery, and the risk involved with pessaries is minimal. Given this risk/benefit ratio, which favors the use of pessaries, it behooves health care professionals to offer the continence pessary as a first option to all women with pure stress or mixed incontinence.

KEY POINTS
1. Stress urinary incontinence, leaking of urine with coughing, laughing, and physical activities, is caused by a failure of the urethral sphincter.
2. Continence pessaries are an effective treatment for stress incontinence, which works well for over 50% of women who are fitted.
3. Continence pessaries work equally well for women with either pure stress incontinence or mixed incontinence.
4. Prior pelvic surgery, particularly incontinence surgery, is associated with higher continence pessary failure.
5. Complications with continence pessaries are minimal.

References
1. Palmer MH. Incontinence: the magnitude of the problem. Nurs Clin North Am 1998;23:139–157.
2. Diokno AC, Brock BM, Brown MB, et al. Prevalence of urinary incontinence and other urologic symptoms in non-institutionalized elderly. J Urol 1986;136:1022–1025.
3. Hørding U, Pedersen K, Sidenius K, et al. Urinary incontinence in 45 year old women. Scand J Urol Nephrol 1986;20:183–186.
4. Hunskaar S, Lose G, Sykes D, Voss S. The prevalence of urinary incontinence in women in four European countries. Br J Urol 2004; 93:324–330.
5. Wilson L, Brown JS, Shin GP, Luc KO, Subak LL. Annual direct cost of urinary incontinence. Obstet Gynecol 2001;98:398–406.
6. Hu TW, Wagner TH, Bentkover JD, Leblanc K, Zhou SZ, Hunt T. Costs of urinary incontinence and overactive bladder in the United States: a comparative study. Urology 2004;63:461–465.
7. Summi HRL, Bent AE. Genuine stress incontinence: an overview. In: Ostergard DR, Bent AE, eds. Urogynecology and Urodynamics: Theory and Practice, 3rd ed. Baltimore: Williams and Wilkins. 1991;393–403.
8. Drutz H, Farrell SA, Mainprize, TC. Guidelines for the evaluation of genuine stress incontinence prior to primary surgery. J Soc Obstet Gynecol Can 1997;19:633–639.
9. Fraser M, Lose G, Kozman E, Boos K, Tincello D. Mechanical devices for urinary incontinence in women (Protocol for Cochrane Review). The Cochrane Library, Issue 2, 2003. Oxford: Update Software.
10. Adams E, Thomson A, Maher C, Hagen S. Mechanical devices for pelvic organ prolapse in women (review). The Cochrane Library, Issue 1, 2004. Oxford: Update Software.
11. Robert M, Mainprize TC. Long term assessment of the incontinence ring pessary for the treatment of stress incontinence. Int Urogynecol J Pelvic Floor Dysfunct 2002;13(5):326–329.
12. Donnelly MJ, Powell-Morgan S, Olsen AL, Nygaard IE. Vaginal pessaries for the management of stress and mixed urinary incontinence. Int Urogynecol J Pelvic Floor Dysfunct 2004;15(5):302–307.
13. Farrell SA, Singh B, Aldakhil L. Continence pessaries in the management of urinary incontinence in women. J Obstet Gynecol Can 2004;26(2):113–117.
14. Clemens JL, Aguilar VC, Tillinghast TA, Jackson ND, Myers DL. Patient satisfaction and changes in prolapse and urinary symptoms in women who are fitted successfully with a pessary for pelvic organ prolapse. Am J Obstet Gynecol 2004;190(4):1025–1029.
15. Bhatia NN, Bergman A, Gunning JE. Urodynamic effect of a vaginal pessary in women with stress urinary incontinence. Am J Obstet Gynecol 1983;147:876–884.
16. Morris AR, Moore KH. The Contiform incontinence device—efficacy and patient acceptability. Int Urogynecol J Pelvic Floor Dysfunct 2003;14(6):412–417.

17. Baydock S, Farrell SA. Effectiveness of uresta self-fitting continence pessary set for women. J Obstet Gynaecol Can 2004;26:S36.
18. Farrell SA. A triage approach to the investigation and management of urinary incontinence. J Soc Obstet Gynecol Can 1998;20:1153–1158.
19. Black N, Griffiths J, Pope C, Bowling A, Abel P. Impact of surgery for stress incontinence on morbidity: a cohort study. BMJ 1997;315: 1493–1498.
20. Bo K, Kvarstein B, Nygaard I. Lower urinary tract symptoms and pelvic floor muscle exercise adherence after 15 years. Obstet Gynecol 2005;105:999–1005.

Chapter 4
Selection of a Patient for Pessary Care

Scott A. Farrell

4.1 OUTLINE

Most women with symptomatic pelvic organ prolapse are candidates for conservative management using a pessary. A comprehensive medical history and physical examination of the pelvis is sufficient assessment. This chapter discusses the following issues:

1. Factors influencing patient selection for a pessary
2. The evaluation undertaken prior to pessary fitting

4.2 INTRODUCTION

Among healthcare professionals who care for women with pelvic prolapse, there is a lack of consensus on the use of pessaries.[1] While most utilize them as a first-line therapy, some believe a pessary should be offered only to individuals who are not candidates for pelvic repair surgery. This bias against the routine use of pessaries is based on the assumption that surgery is preferred by patients[2] and that pessaries are associated with significant risk.[3,4]

Women with pelvic organ prolapse with or without accompanying incontinence should be made aware of the evidence concerning both conservative therapy and surgery. This discussion, if presented in a balanced way, will touch on the long-term effectiveness of pelvic prolapse surgery[5] and the potential risks and complications of this surgery.[6] Pessaries should be presented as an effective alternative with few risks and complications but requiring an adjustment of lifestyle. Women who are more likely to opt for a pessary include (1) those who are older,[7,8] (2) those with greater degrees of pelvic prolapse,[7] and (3) those who have no choice because of medical contraindications to surgery.[9]

4.3 EVALUATION OF THE PATIENT PRIOR TO PESSARY FITTING

The evaluation of the patient should include a complete history of pelvic function (Table 4.1) and a past medical history (Table 4.2). Examination should include a general physical examination and a careful pelvic examination. The latter has as its goals (1) quantification of the extent of pelvic support defects in the anterior (bladder), apical (uterus/vaginal vault), and posterior (rectum) compartments (Figure 4.1); (2) assessment of the

TABLE 4.1. History of pelvic function in a patient with pelvic prolapse

General pelvic symptoms
    Pelvic pressure and pain
    Palpable or visible tissue at the introitus
    Dyspareunia
    Interference with mobility and function

Urinary tract symptoms
Obstructive symptoms
    Frequency
    Incomplete emptying
    Urgency/urgency incontinence
Stress incontinence: Current or prior history

Gastrointestinal tract
    Incontinence of flatus or feces
    Difficult rectal evacuation
    Splinting

TABLE 4.2. Past medical history of patient with pelvic prolapse

General medical health and medications
Sexual activity
Prior treatment of prolapse
Surgical care: Number and type of pelvic surgical procedures
Medical care
    Hormone replacement
    Medical management of urinary tract symptoms
Pessaries
    Types and sizes used
    Reason for pessary failure

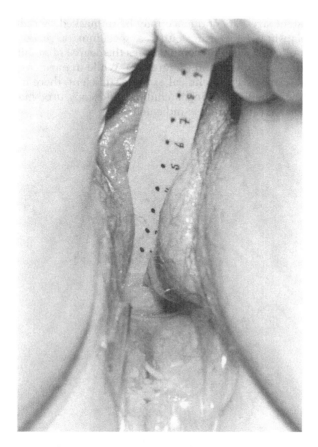

FIGURE 4.1. Pelvic organ prolapse quantification (POP-Q) of the extent of pelvic prolapse. (From Farrell SA. Clinical evaluation of the pelvis. In: Drutz HP, Herschorn S, Diamant NE, eds. Female Pelvic Medicine and Reconstructive Pelvic Surgery. London: Springer-Verlag, 2003:85. With Kind permission of Springer Science and Business Media.)

integrity of the perineal body; (3) determination of the health of the vaginal epithelium (thickness and evidence of abnormal discharge); (4) quantification of the strength of the pelvic muscles; (5) assessment of the length and caliber of the vaginal canal; and (6) estimation of the angle formed between the inferior pubic rami. In patients with more severe degrees of pelvic organ prolapse, latent stress incontinence may be unmasked by reducing the prolapsing tissue using either a speculum or rectal swab (Figure 4.2). Q-tip testing demonstrates the degree of mobility of the urethrovesical junction (Figure 4.3). While in most cases the above-described careful clinical exam is sufficient, there may be cases where ancillary testing, including endoscopy, urodynamics, and endoanal ultrasound, is indicated.

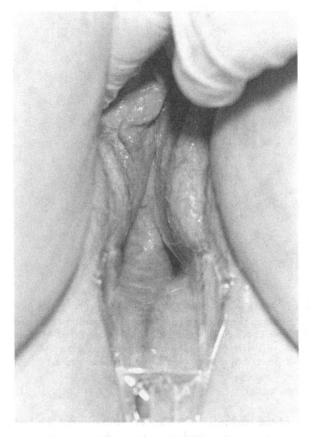

FIGURE 4.2. A speculum is used to look at the anterior vaginal wall and may unmask latent stress incontinence. (From Farrell SA. Clinical evaluation of the pelvis. In: Drutz HP, Herschorn S, Diamant NE, eds. Female Pelvic Medicine and Reconstructive Pelvic Surgery. London: Springer-Verlag, 2003:89. With Kind permission of Springer Science and Business Media.)

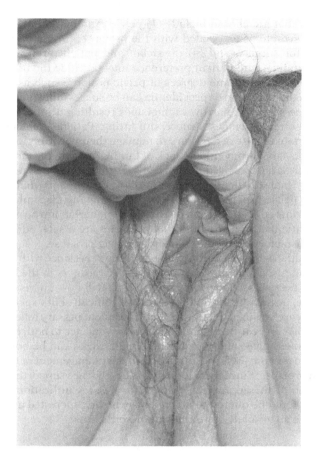

FIGURE 4.3. A Q-tip test is performed. (From Farrell SA. Clinical evaluation of the pelvis. In: Drutz HP, Herschorn S, Diamant NE, eds. Female Pelvic Medicine and Reconstructive Pelvic Surgery. London: Springer-Verlag, 2003:88. With Kind permission of Springer Science and Business Media.)

4.4 DEVELOPING A MANAGEMENT PLAN

Contraindications to a pessary fitting include (1) undiagnosed vaginal discharge, (2) undiagnosed vaginal bleeding, (3) acute pelvic inflammatory disease, (4) a noncompliant patient who is likely to be lost to follow-up, and (5) a lack of assured follow-up.[10]

Once the patient evaluation is completed, a management plan that includes both conservative and surgical alternatives can be discussed with the patient. Factors influencing the management options that are chosen include (1) pelvic examination findings, (2) the symptoms associated with the prolapse, (3) the patient's fitness for surgery, and (4) physician and patient preferences. Pelvic findings and patient preference may preclude the use of a pessary.[8] While extreme degrees of pelvic prolapse such as complete vaginal eversion or procidentia can be successfully managed with a pessary,[11,12] a narrow vaginal apex resulting from previous surgery often precludes a successful fitting. Patients' reluctance to entertain the use of a pessary to manage their pelvic organ prolapse may arise from either a lack of familiarity with pessaries or misinformation received from friends. Before seeing the modern pessary, many patients imagine archaic instruments that may correct pelvic prolapse but at the cost of ongoing discomfort. If appropriate educational and instructional materials are provided, most patients can be assured that pessaries are a safe, effective, and satisfactory method of managing pelvic prolapse.

Healthcare professionals who have little experience with using pessaries are daunted by prospects of awkwardness in the handling of pessaries and troublesome frequent follow-up visits. In practice, pessary fitting and care is not a difficult skill to acquire, and research evidence confirms that convenient pessary follow-up protocols can be used that minimize inconvenience to both health care professionals and the patients.[11,12] Pessaries can be both an effective and the preferred approach to the management of pelvic organ prolapse. Since there is no scientific evidence supporting the selection of the appropriate patient for pessary utilization, pessaries should be offered to all patients who are interested and do not have an absolute contraindication to their use.

4.5 SUMMARY AND REVIEW OF KEY POINTS
In this chapter, the appropriate evaluation of a patient with pelvic organ prolapse was discussed. Factors that should be considered in developing a management plan were outlined.

KEY POINTS
1. Pessaries should be offered to all patients with symptomatic pelvic organ prolapse.
2. The evaluation of women prior to pessary fitting should be comprehensive without involving complex and invasive tests.
3. Most patients are candidates for a trial of a pessary.
4. Fitting and management of pessaries can be simplified and routinized to minimize inconvenience to both health care professionals and patients.

References

1. Cundiff GW, Weidner AC, Visco AG, Bump RC, Addison WA. A survey of pessary use by members of the American Urogynecologic Society. Obstet Gynecol 2000;95:931–935.
2. Bash KL. Review of vaginal pessaries. Obstet Gynecol Surv 2000; 55:455–460.
3. Mueller-Heubach E. A pessary can be dangerous. J Med Soc N J 1970; 67:104–106.
4. Russel JK. The dangerous pessary. BMJ 1961;2:1595–1597.
5. Olsen A, Smith VJ, Bergstrom JO, Colling JC, Clark AL. Epidemiology of surgically managed pelvic organ prolapse and urinary incontinence. Obstet Gynecol 1997;89:501–506.
6. Brown JS, Waetjen LE, Subak LL, Thom DH, Van Den Eeden S, Vittinghoff E. Pelvic organ prolapse surgery in the United States, 1997. Am J Obstet Gynecol 2004;186:712–716.
7. Heit M, Rosenquist C, Culligan P, Graham C, Murphy M, Shott S. Predicting treatment choice for patients with pelvic organ prolapse. Obstet Gynecol 2003;101:1279–1284.
8. Clemons J, Aguilar VC, Sokol ER, Jackson ND, Myers DL. Patient characteristics that are associated with continued pessary use versus surgery after 1 year. Am J Obstet Gynecol 2004;191:159–164.
9. Bai SW, Yoon BS, Kwon JY, Shin JS, Kim SK, Park KH. Survey of the characteristics and satisfaction degree of the patients using a pessary. Int Urogynecol J 2005;16:182–186.
10. Miller DS. Contemporary use of the pessary. In: Doegmueller W, Sciarra JJ, eds. Gynecology and Obstetrics, vol 1. Philadelphia: Lippincott-Raven, 1991;1–12.
11. Clemons JL, Aguilar VC, Tillinghast TA, Jackson ND, Myers DL. Risk factors associated with an unsuccessful pessary fitting trial in women with pelvic organ prolapse. Am J Obstet Gynecol 2003;190:345–350.
12. Wu V, Farrell SA, Baskett TF, Flowerdew G. A simplified protocol for pessary management. Obstet Gynecol 1997;90:990–904.

Chapter 5

Selection of Pessaries for Pelvic Organ Prolapse

Sandra A. Baydock and Scott A. Farrell

5.1 OUTLINE

The selection of a pessary to treat pelvic prolapse has traditionally been based on the practitioners clinical experience and the
received wisdom of mentors. Guidelines from manufacturers are
not based on scientific evidence but rather on the recommendations of the inventors and those of recognized authorities. Clinical research has provided some guidance. This chapter discusses
the following issues:

1. The use of clinical evidence along with pragmatic considerations to provide a new and more effective rationale for pessary
   selection
2. The features of the most commonly used pessaries, and the
   impact these features have on pessary selection

5.2 INTRODUCTION

All pessaries described in this chapter are made of medical-grade
silicone with the exception of the Inflatoball, which is made of
latex rubber. Silicone has several advantages over other materials.
It is inert and therefore has very low allergenicity. It does not
absorb secretions and thus reduces the likelihood of experiencing
vaginal odor during pessary use. Finally, silicone pessaries can be
autoclaved and are resistant to degradation by most antiseptics.[1]
Pessaries discarded during a pessary fitting trial can be sterilized
for reuse, thus decreasing the cost to both provider and patient.

Pessaries for pelvic organ prolapse are arbitrarily divided into
two categories: support pessaries and space-occupying pessaries.[2]
Support pessaries include the ring, ring with support, Gehrung,
and lever pessaries (Figure 5.1). They lie along the vaginal axis,
with the posterior component sitting in the posterior vaginal
fornix and the anterior component coming to rest just under the

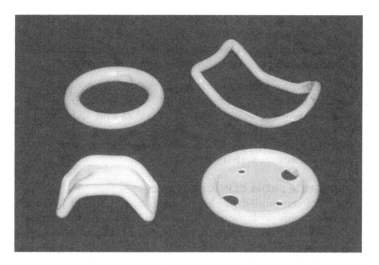

FIGURE 5.1. Examples of support pessaries: open ring, ring with support, Gehrung, and Hodge.

symphysis pubis. These pessaries therefore create a "supportive shelf." Space-occupying pessaries include the Gellhorn, cube, donut, and Inflatoball (Figure 5.2). Their support effect results from their impingement on surrounding structures in the pelvis.

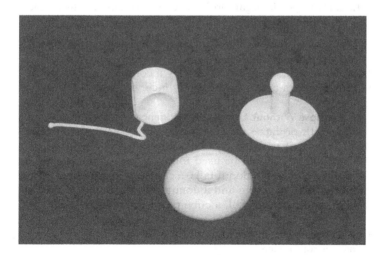

FIGURE 5.2. Examples of space-occupying pessaries: Gellhorn, cube, and donut.

Given the scant amount of research evidence available to guide pessary selection, clinical practice must be guided for the most part by pragmatic considerations. The recommendations in this chapter are based on the following considerations:

1. Evidence from limited clinical trials[1,3–6]
2. Clinical indications for pessary use
3. The feasibility of easy insertion, removal, and self-care with different pessary models
4. Potential complications with different pessary models
5. Desire for sexual activity by the patient

5.3 EVIDENCE FROM CLINICAL TRIALS

A review of the published clinical trials on the use of pessaries for pelvic organ prolapse reveals a very consistent pattern (see Chapter 3). With the exception of one study,[1] the authors chose to try a ring pessary as the first-line pessary for pelvic organ prolapse. When the ring pessary failed, or in the view of the authors was not indicated, then the Gellhorn pessary was used as a second option. Where the Gellhorn pessary failed, the cube pessary was most often tried as the third option. While most authors referred to the use of other pessaries on occasion, the ring, Gellhorn, and cube were most commonly used.

5.4 CLINICAL INDICATIONS FOR PESSARY USE

Patients with pelvic organ prolapse can be pragmatically divided into the following groups:

1. Prolapse without either concurrent or latent stress urinary incontinence
2. Prolapse with latent stress urinary incontinence
3. Prolapse with concurrent urinary incontinence

5.4.1 Prolapse Without Urinary Incontinence

Women with prolapse unaccompanied by urinary incontinence should be fitted with an ordinary ring pessary. When the ring fails, a Gellhorn should be used followed by a donut pessary if the Gellhorn fails. If a donut fails, a combination of either a ring and a Gellhorn or a ring and a donut pessary should be tried. If combination pessaries fail, a cube pessary should be used.

5.4.2 Prolapse with Either Latent or Concurrent Urinary Incontinence

Women who have prolapse with associated latent stress urinary incontinence will experience an unmasking of their incontinence if the prolapse is reduced using a pessary that does not support the urethra. For that reason, the ring pessary with support and knob is the logical first choice for these women. If the ring with knob is unsuccessful, a Gellhorn, in some cases, can restore support to both the prolapse and the urethra, thus preventing incontinence. If the Gellhorn is unsuccessful, a cube pessary may also be used in these patients. It should be inserted so that one of the edges of the cube is placed strategically beneath the urethra.[7]

The above approach should work equally well for women who complain of both prolapse and urinary incontinence.

5.5 FEASIBILITY OF PESSARY USE (BOTH PATIENT AND PHYSICIAN COMFORT)

Pessary design features have a significant impact on both patient and physician ease of use and comfort with pessaries. In the following sections the relevant features of the most popular pessaries are discussed. An algorithm for the selection of a pessary for pelvic prolapse is shown in Figure 5.3.

5.5.1 Ring Pessary

The ring pessary has been used successfully to treat all types and degrees of pelvic prolapse and should be the first choice for a woman with prolapse of any degree (Figure 5.4). The ring pessary is made of solid silicone in which are embedded two plastic semicircular inserts. These inserts increase the rigidity of the pessary sides while permitting the pessary to be made of a very flexible silicone. The ring pessary is the easiest pessary for women to use and for health care providers to prescribe. It is relatively easy to grasp and remove, and for this reason patients are more likely to be able to manage this pessary themselves. It is the only pessary designed to treat pelvic prolapse that can be folded. Folding the pessary significantly reduces its size and allows for easier introduction through the vaginal introitus. The ring pessary sits along the vaginal axis and does not sequester vaginal secretions, which degenerate and produce odor. Intercourse is possible with this pessary. The open ring comes in 14 sizes from small (0) to large (13), ranging in diameter from 44 to 127 mm. The ring with support is available in 15 sizes ranging from small (0) to large (14).

5.5.2 Gellhorn Pessary

The Gellhorn pessary has been used successfully to treat all degrees of prolapse but it is preferentially used to treat higher

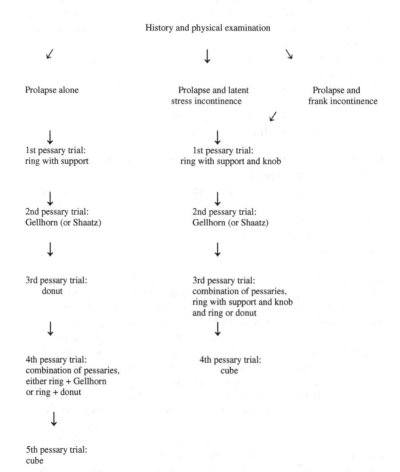

Guidelines for Pessary Selection

History and physical examination

Prolapse alone

Prolapse and latent
stress incontinence

Prolapse and
frank incontinence

1st pessary trial:
ring with support

1st pessary trial:
ring with support and knob

2nd pessary trial:
Gellhorn (or Shaatz)

2nd pessary trial:
Gellhorn (or Shaatz)

3rd pessary trial:
donut

3rd pessary trial:
combination of pessaries,
ring with support and knob
and ring or donut

4th pessary trial:
combination of pessaries,
either ring + Gellhorn
or ring + donut

4th pessary trial:
cube

5th pessary trial:
cube

FIGURE 5.3. Algorithm for the selection of a pessary for pelvic prolapse.

stages of uterine or vaginal apical prolapse (Figure 5.5). Its
design makes it more difficult to handle for both health care professionals and women. The Gellhorn pessary is solid and is made
of either flexible or rigid silicone or rigid acrylic. The base is circular with a concave surface on the bottom and a convex surface
on the top to which is affixed, at its midpoint, a column of varying
lengths ending in a knob. The circular base is perforated at

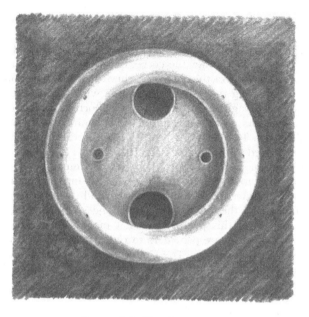

FIGURE 5.4. The ring pessary.

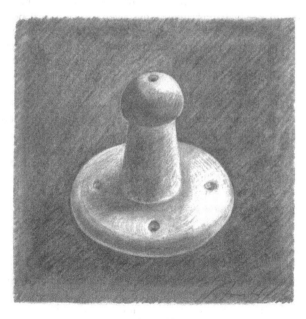

FIGURE 5.5. The Gellhorn pessary.

regular intervals by holes and the column by a central hole to allow drainage of vaginal secretions. When the Gellhorn is inserted, its concave surface sits at a 90-degree angle to the vaginal axis against either the cervix or the vaginal vault and it exerts a suction effect that helps pessary retention. The column comes to lie along the axis of the vagina with the knob sitting just inside the vaginal introitus. The Gellhorn is available in a version that has a shorter column to fit women with shorter vaginal length. The Gellhorn pessary has several disadvantages when compared to the ring pessary. It cannot be folded to reduce its size for vaginal insertion. The pessary must be inserted perpendicular to the floor and the vaginal introitus must be depressed in order to get the pessary beyond the inferior pubic rami that guard the vaginal introitus. The suction action and bulkier nature of this pessary make it more difficult for both women and health care providers to remove. Intercourse is not possible with this pessary. The Gellhorn pessary comes in nine sizes ranging from small with a 38-mm (1.5-inch) diameter base to large with an 89-mm (3.5-inch) base.

5.5.3 Shaatz Pessary

There are no published data on the use of the Shaatz pessary (Figure 5.6). It is essentially a Gellhorn pessary without the column and knob. It has advantages over the Gellhorn because it doesn"t have a column and it can be folded, though not as completely as the ring pessary, for insertion through the vaginal introitus. However, removal of the Shaatz is more difficult than both the ring and Gellhorn pessaries because it does not fold as completely as the ring and lacks the Gellhorn knob. Like the Gellhorn, the Shaatz probably functions as a space-occupying pessary with some suction effect. Because it lacks the central column and knob, it will tend to come to rest along the vaginal axis in a similar orientation to the ring pessary. The Shaatz pessary may be indicated in women who would normally be fitted with a Gellhorn but who prefer not to handle the pessary themselves and are interested in preserving the possibility of intercourse. The Shaatz pessary is available in the same sizes as the Gellhorn.

5.5.4 Donut Pessary

The donut pessary is thought to be a very popular option among health care professionals, although it is not reported in any of the clinical trial publications (Figure 5.7). It is shaped very similarly to the inner tube of a tire. Its height is significantly greater

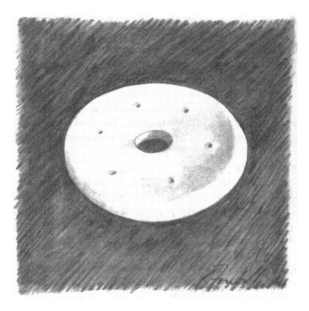

FIGURE 5.6. The Shaatz pessary.

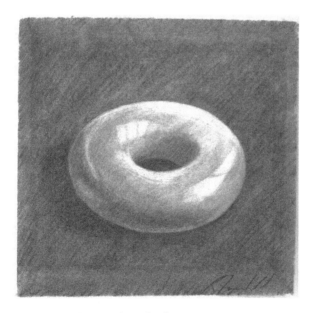

FIGURE 5.7. The donut pessary.

than that of the ring pessary and although it is soft, its shape and size cannot be modified significantly to permit easy insertion into and removal from the vagina. The donut shares some of the advantages of the ring pessary. It will not sequester vaginal secretions and it is inserted directly into the vagina without any additional manipulation. Because its size cannot be reduced, it may cause significant discomfort during insertion and removal. Intercourse is not possible with this pessary. The donut pessary comes in eight sizes ranging from a small of 51 mm to a large of 95 mm.

5.5.5 Cube Pessary

The cube pessary is highly effective at treating apical vaginal vault prolapse that is unresponsive to the ring and Gellhorn (Figure 5.8). While the cube may be used successfully when all other types of pessaries have failed, its drawbacks are significant and include a higher predisposition to vaginal erosions, the need for daily removal to avoid vaginal odor, and a general difficulty with both insertion and removal.

The cube pessary is comprised of six concave surfaces that interact like suction cups with the surrounding vaginal wall. It is

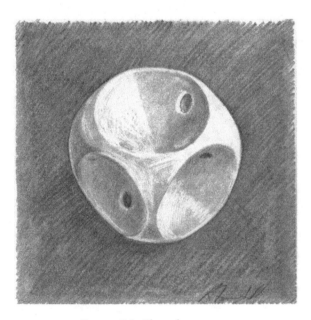

FIGURE 5.8. The cube pessary.

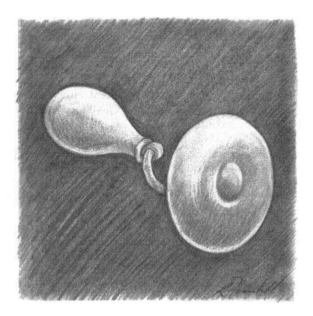

FIGURE 5.9. The Inflatoball pessary.

a space-filling pessary that acts by both its bulk and by its suction action. The ridges between the concave surfaces are somewhat narrow and sharp and tend to cause vaginal erosions. Because this pessary tends to sequester vaginal secretions, it should be removed on a daily basis. A model with perforations that permit drainage of vaginal secretions is available. This modification means that the pessary can be left in the vagina for longer periods of time. The cube pessary is extremely difficult to manipulate for insertion. The best description we can offer is that it must be "scrunched" in order to reduce its size for insertion. The cube pessary comes in eight sizes ranging from small (0) to large (7) and measuring 25 to 57 mm.

5.5.6 Inflatoball

The Inflatoball has a shape very similar to that of the donut pessary. It has the advantage that it can be deflated for easier insertion into the vagina (Figure 5.9). After insertion the pessary is pumped up and the inflation tubing is tucked into the vagina. Because this pessary is made of latex it cannot be used by women with latex allergies. It also tends to absorb vaginal secretions and therefore must be removed and cleaned on a daily basis. The inflatoball comes in four sizes from small at 51 mm to extra large at 70 mm.

5.5.7 Gehrung Pessary

The Gehrung pessary was designed to treat either a cystocele or rectocele (Figure 5.10). It is an arch-shaped pessary with arms that can be manually shaped. Insertion and removal of this pessary is very difficult. Because this pessary has never been tested for clinical efficacy and anecdotal evidence would suggest that it is infrequently used in the management of pelvic organ prolapse, it is unlikely to be of much value clinically. The Gehrung comes in 10 sizes ranging from small (0) to large (9).

5.5.8 Lever Pessaries (Smith, Hodge, and Risser)

Lever pessaries have traditionally been used for the treatment of uterine retroversion (Figure 5.11). Several case reports and expert articles have been written about their use for this indica-

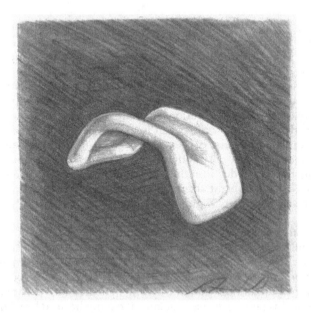

FIGURE 5.10. The Gehrung pessary.

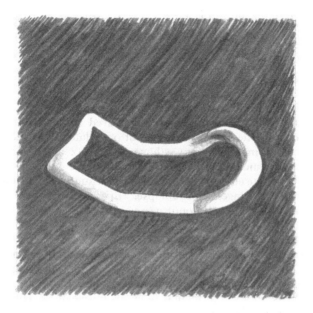

FIGURE 5.11. The Hodge pessary, a lever-type pessary.

tion during the last century.[8–10] Since uterine retroversion is usually asymptomatic in the nonpregnant state, the lever pessary is rarely used for this indication in modern gynecology. During pregnancy, uterine retroversion may produce pelvic discomfort, and when it is complicated by uterine incarceration it becomes an obstetrical emergency. If the uterus can be successfully anteverted, the lever pessary can be used to keep it in that position until it moves out of the pelvis in the second trimester.

The lever pessaries that are most commonly used are the Smith, Hodge, and Risser. Lever pessaries have an S-shaped configuration with a wide concave posterior component that comes to rest in the posterior fornix behind the uterus, and a convex anterior portion that comes in various shapes depending on the particular lever pessary. The anterior portion of the Smith is rounded, the Hodge is rectangular, and the Risser has a wider, rectangular anterior arch with an indentation. One version of the Hodge pessary comes with a covered anterior component meant for patients with associated cystocele. The Risser has a wider anterior bar and deeper notch designed to create a larger weight-bearing surface along the anterior component. Intercourse should be possible with lever pessaries. The Hodge pessary comes in 10 sizes. The Smith pessary comes in nine sizes and the Risser comes in 10 sizes.

5.5.9 Double Pessaries

In patients with more severe stages of pelvic prolapse, single pessaries may fail. In these cases a trial of double pessaries is warranted. Two small case series achieved success with this approach.[11,12] One series used a donut or Inflatoball as the lead pessary combined with a Gellhorn or Shaatz as the second pessary with success in five patients with stage 4 prolapse.[11] A second report used two ring pessaries with success in 13 out of 18 women with stage 3 or 4 prolapse.[12] In our experience, a combination of the ring and donut pessary has worked well.

5.6 POTENTIAL FOR COMPLICATIONS

Common complications encountered with pessaries include vaginal discharge, odor, vaginal erosion, vaginal bleeding, and discomfort.[1,4] All of these complications can be minimized when a pessary is removed at regular intervals for cleaning. This care is most practically done by the woman who is using the pessary. For this reason, pessaries that are most easily inserted and removed by the patient should be used whenever possible. For women who do not take care of their pessary, it is preferable to use a pessary that is less likely to trap secretions such as the ring, Shaatz, or donut pessaries. The likelihood of vaginal erosions is highest using the cube pessary because of its sharp edges.[4] Pessaries that are too large also cause pressure erosions.

5.7 DESIRE FOR SEXUAL ACTIVITY

It is not possible to have sexual intercourse when any of the space-occupying pessaries is in the vagina. These pessaries include the Gellhorn, cube, donut, and Inflatoball. Some patients are able to have vaginal intercourse while using support pessaries such as the ring, Shaatz, lever, and Gehrung pessaries, although there is no published clinical evidence that this is possible.

5.8 SUMMARY AND REVIEW OF KEY POINTS

This chapter discussed the factors, both scientific and pragmatic, that when taken into consideration provide the basis for a logical approach to the selection of a pessary. The design features of the most effective and frequently used pessaries have been described and potential pessary-related complications outlined.

KEY POINTS

1. Most pessaries are made of medical-grade silicone or rubber, which does not absorb secretions or cause allergic reactions.
2. Two general categories of pessaries are the support type and the space-occupying type.
3. Published clinical trials of pessaries have used the following order for trying pessaries: ring, Gellhorn, cube, and other.
4. The presence of urinary incontinence in association with pelvic prolapse mandates the use of pessaries that support the urethra.
5. The ring pessary is the most universally acceptable and practical pessary for pelvic organ prolapse.

References

1. Sulak PJ, Kuehl TJ, Shull BL. Vaginal pessaries and their use in pelvic relaxation. J Reprod Med 1993;38(12):919–923.
2. Cundiff GW, Weidner AC, Visco AG, Bump RC, Addison WA. A survey of pessary use by members of the American Urogynecology Society. Obstet Gynecol 2000;95(6):931–935.
3. Clemons JL, Aguilar VC, Tillinghast TA, Jackson ND, Myers DL. Risk factors associated with an unsuccessful pessary fitting trial in women with pelvic organ prolapse. Am J Obstet Gynecol 2004;190:345–350.
4. Wu V, Farrell SA, Baskett TF, Flowerdew G. A simplified protocol for pessary management. Obstet Gynecol 1997;90:990–994.
5. Hanson LM, Schulz JA, Flood GC, Cooley B, Tam F. Vaginal pessaries in managing women with pelvic organ prolapse and urinary incontinence: patient characteristics and factors contributing to success. Int Urogynecol J 2006;17(2):155–159.
6. Bai SW, Yoon BS, Kwon JY, Shin JS, Kim SK, Park KH. Survey of the characteristics and satisfaction degree of the patients using a pessary. Int Urogynecol J 2005;16:182–186.
7. Farrell SA. Pessaries for the management of stress urinary incontinence. J Obstet Gynaecol Can 2001;23:1184–1189.
8. Dreger RB, Menzin AW, Mikuta JJ. The vaginal pessary: past and present. Postgrad Obstet Gynecol 1993;13:1–7.
9. Zeitlin MP, Lebherz TB. Pessaries in the geriatric patient. J Am Geriatr Soc 1992;40:635–640.
10. Poma PA. Nonsurgical management of genital prolapse; a review and recommendations for clinical practice. J Reprod Med 2000;45:789–797.
11. Myers DL, LaSala CA, Murphy JA. Double pessary use in grade 4 uterine and vaginal prolapse. Obstet Gynecol 1998;91:1019–1020.
12. Singh K, Reid WM. Non-surgical treatment of uterovaginal prolapse using double vaginal rings. Br J Obstet Gynaecol 2002;109:1427.

Chapter 6
Selection of Pessaries for Urinary Incontinence

Baharak Amir-Khalkhali and Scott A. Farrell

6.1 OUTLINE
Although a large number of pessaries are purportedly designed to treat urinary incontinence, only a few pessaries have actually undergone clinical trial. This chapter discusses the qualities of the most commonly used continence pessaries and indications for their use. This chapter discusses the following issues:

1. Categories of continence pessaries
2. The design features of continence pessaries and the impact these features have on pessary selection

6.2 INTRODUCTION
Continence pessaries work in the same way as surgery, by providing mechanical support to the urethra.[1] The majority of pessaries designed specifically to treat urinary incontinence are equipped with a knob that must be positioned in the midline of the vagina under the urethra in order to provide this mechanical support. These pessaries include the incontinence ring (Figure 6.1), the ring pessary with knob (Figure 6.2), and the incontinence dish (Figure 6.3). Other pessaries, whose primary purpose is to correct uterine retrodisplacement or rectocele, have also been equipped with incontinence knobs by some manufacturers. There are two pessary designs that depart from the others in their design, the Mar-land pessary (Mentor Corp, Santa Barbara, California, USA) (Figure 6.4) and the Urestra pessary (EastMed Inc., Halifax, Nova Scotia, Canada) (Figure 6.5). As discussed in Chapter 3, there is very little evidence in the medical literature concerning the effectiveness of most continence pessaries, with the exception of the incontinence ring, the ring with support and knob, and the Urestra pessaries.[2-5] In our clinical experience, these pessaries are used most frequently to treat urinary incontinence and should be the first-line choices.

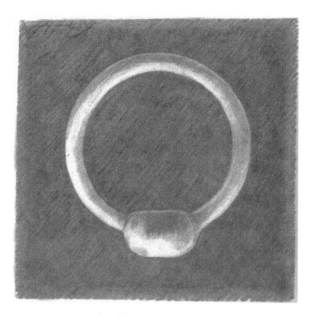

FIGURE 6.1. The incontinence ring pessary.

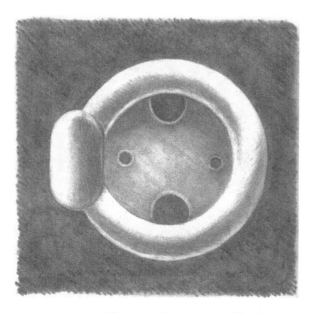

FIGURE 6.2. The ring with support and knob.

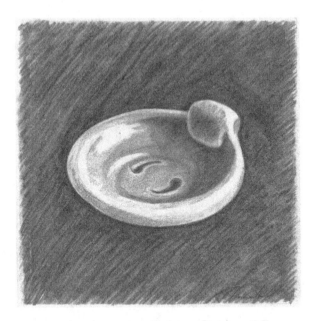

FIGURE 6.3. The incontinence dish pessary.

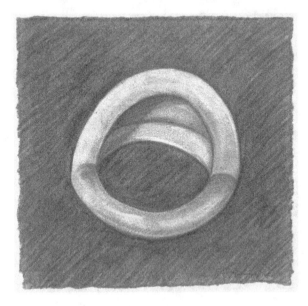

FIGURE 6.4. The Mar-land pessary.

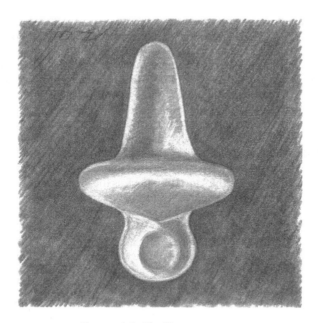

FIGURE 6.5. The Uresta pessary.

6.3 TYPES OF CONTINENCE PESSARIES
Continence pessaries can be divided into three groups based on their design and mechanism of action:

1. Urethral support with a knob: Incontinence ring
2. Urethral support with a knob and cystocele support: Ring with support and knob, incontinence dish
3. Urethral support with bell-shape: Uresta

6.3.1 Incontinence Ring
Both healthcare professionals and women can easily insert the incontinence ring pessary because it is flexible and is inserted directly into the vagina along the posterior vaginal wall. However, its flexibility is also its shortcoming because the ring is not rigid enough to provide effective support of a significant cystocele. For this reason it tends to be displaced and becomes ineffective when a cystocele accompanies stress incontinence. It is most useful for patients complaining of stress urinary incontinence without pelvic organ prolapse. The incontinence ring can be left in place during intercourse. The incontinence ring comes in sizes ranging from small (0) to large (10).

6.3.2 Ring Pessary with Knob

The ring pessary with knob is a heavier, more rigid pessary of the same design as the standard ring pessary. As a result, it can be used to treat both cystocele and urinary incontinence. It is the logical choice for a patient in whom the incontinence ring has been expelled by Valsalva maneuvers. This pessary is more difficult to insert and position because it must be folded (like the ring pessary) for insertion, and the knob must be rotated into position beneath the urethra after the pessary is inserted. For removal, it must be rotated to the side and flexed as it comes out. Some women are able to leave this pessary in the vagina during intercourse. The ring with support and knob has the same drawback as the incontinence ring—problems with displacement of the knob. The ring with support and knob comes in sizes ranging from small (0) to large (10).

6.3.3 Uresta Continence Pessary

The Uresta pessary is the first pessary to be made available to women over the counter. This pessary comes in five sizes from small (2) to large (6). It is provided to initial users as a set of three pessaries, sizes 3, 4, and 5. This pessary kit is accompanied by a pessary-carrying compact and instructions for self-fitting and care (Figure 6.6). The Uresta pessary is designed to be

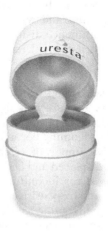

FIGURE 6.6. Uresta pessary in its carrying compact.

inserted directly into the vagina and, like a tampon, to fall naturally into place with the wide base of the bell sitting under the urethra to provide support. Rotation of the pessary along its axis does not displace this support. The handle facilitates insertion and removal of the pessary. While this pessary must be removed for intercourse, the ease with which women handle it means that it will not interfere with sexual activity.

6.3.4 Incontinence Dish

The incontinence dish is very similar in design to the ring with knob. It is intended to be used when a cystocele accompanies stress incontinence. Because it lacks the rigid plastic arms of the ring pessary it can be folded like the incontinence ring for direct insertion into the vagina. It is more likely, however, that this pessary will get hung up in front of the cervix during insertion, thereby displacing the knob away from the urethra so that it will fail to provide effective support. Intercourse may be possible with this pessary in place.

6.3.5 Other Continence Pessaries

Although a number of other pessaries have been modified by the addition of a knob to support the urethra and stop urinary incontinence, there has been no research conducted to assess their effectiveness. The design of the Mar-land pessary makes it extremely difficult to fold and manipulate for insertion and removal.

6.4 OTHER PESSARY ALTERNATIVES FOR STRESS INCONTINENCE

We have used both the cube and Gellhorn pessaries to successfully treat stress incontinence.[1] They are particularly effective when previous surgery has narrowed the vaginal caliber or reduced the urethral mobility. The cube pessary can be positioned so that one of its ridges sits beneath and at right angles to the urethra. A model that has perforations to allow vaginal secretions to drain is preferable because it can be left in place for a longer period of time. The Gellhorn pessary can also be positioned so that the wide base of the pessary sits under the urethra, elevating and supporting it.

6.5 GUIDELINES FOR SELECTION OF A CONTINENCE PESSARY

When selecting a continence pessary, the health care professional should consider both ease of handling and likelihood of misplacement of the supportive portion away from the urethra. The

Uresta continence pessary has a handle that makes insertion easy. When inserted directly into the vagina, it falls naturally into place and supports the urethra despite rotation along its axis. For these reasons it should be the first choice among continence pessaries. The incontinence ring pessary is flexible and relatively easy to insert because it is inserted directly into the vagina. It should be the second choice. When a cystocele accompanies incontinence, the incontinence dish can be tried because it is easier to insert than the ring with support and knob. If the incontinence dish is ineffective, the ring with support and knob should be used. If all of the above pessaries fail, it may be possible to achieve continence using an alternative pessary such as the Gellhorn or cube.

6.6 SUMMARY AND REVIEW OF KEY POINTS
Only a few pessaries have been specifically designed and tested for the treatment of stress urinary incontinence. This chapter provided a description of the design features of these continence pessaries and a rationale for their selection.

KEY POINTS
1. Several continence pessaries have been proven to effectively treat urinary incontinence.
2. The most important features of a continence pessary are ease of insertion and removal and likelihood of displacement of the support away from the urethra.
3. The Uresta pessary is easiest to insert and most likely to be properly placed.
4. The incontinence dish or the ring with support and knob are most likely to effectively treat both a cystocele and stress incontinence.

References
1. Farrell SA. Pessaries for the management of stress urinary incontinence. J Obstet Gynaecol Can 2001;23:1184–1189.
2. Robert M, Mainprize TC. Long term assessment of the incontinence ring pessary for the treatment of stress incontinence. Int Urogynecol J Pelvic Floor Dysfunct 2002;13:326–329.
3. Donnelly MJ, Powell-Morgan S, Olsen AL, Nygaard IE. Vaginal pessaries for the management of stress and mixed urinary incontinence. Int Urogynecol J Pelvic Floor Dysfunct 2004;15: 302–307.

4. Farrell SA, Singh B, Aldakhil L. Continence pessaries in the management of urinary incontinence in women. J Obstet Gynaecol Can 2004;26:113–117.
5. Baydock S, Farrell SA. Effectiveness of the Uresta™ self-fitting continence pessary set. J Obstet Gynaecol Can 2004;5(suppl):s36.

Chapter 7

Fitting and Care of Pessaries for Pelvic Organ Prolapse

Sandra A. Baydock and Scott A. Farrell

7.1 OUTLINE

The successful management of pelvic organ prolapse with pessaries requires a familiarity and comfort with a variety of pessaries. Each pessary type has unique characteristics that require different approaches to insertion, removal, and care. This chapter discusses the following issues:

1. Preparation of the patient for pessary fitting
2. The fitting and care of the following pessaries:
   a. Ring
   b. Gellhorn
   c. Cube
   d. Donut
   e. Lever

7.2 PREPARATIONS FOR PESSARY FITTING

The trial-and-error process of pessary fitting requires that an array of basic pessary types and sizes be available. The minimum pessary armamentarium should include the ring, ring with support, Gellhorn, donut, and cube pessaries in a range of sizes. The pessaries can be kept in a cart that can be conveniently wheeled into the examination room. The patient should be examined and fitted in the dorsal lithotomy position. Her bladder need not be empty but she should be comfortable. It is preferable that the patient has some urine in her bladder since she should undergo a trial of voiding before leaving the clinic.

7.3 PELVIC EXAMINATION AND PESSARY SIZING

The examination should begin with observation of the vaginal introitus and perineum at rest. Prolapse of a moderate or greater degree will usually be visible on inspection at rest. The patient should then be asked to strain maximally in an effort to reproduce the full extent of the prolapse. Using the blades of a Graves speculum, the anterior, apical, and posterior compartments should be examined in turn. The location and extent of the prolapse should be determined and recorded. The health of the vagina should be noted, with particular attention to vaginal thickness and evidence of erosions or excoriations. A Pap smear should be performed if indicated. A bimanual exam at rest and with straining provides further information about the nature and extent of the prolapse and permits the detection of pelvic masses. The prolapse should be reduced manually before inserting the pessary. In the lithotomy position, the prolapse will often remain reduced for a short period of time, allowing pessary insertion.

The initial pessary type and size should be determined by pelvic exam. The pessary size is determined in two steps. First, by manual examination of the vagina the length of the vagina from the posterior fornix to the symphysis pubis is determined. Second, the vaginal width or caliber is gauged by spreading the index and middle fingers horizontally at the level of the cervix or vaginal vault. A combination of the measurements of vaginal length and vaginal diameter at the apex permits selection of the appropriate pessary size.

7.4 PESSARY INSERTION AND TESTING
A pair of dry gloves should be used with every attempted pessary insertion to ensure that the pessary is controlled. A small amount of lubricant can be placed on the leading edge of the pessary to facilitate insertion. Pessaries provided by the manufacturer are coated in cornstarch and should be rinsed with tap water before use. After insertion of a pessary the patient should be asked to perform a Valsalva maneuver to test its effectiveness. The patient should not feel the pessary if it is properly sized. With most pessaries it should be possible to rock the pessary gently and to insert a finger between the pessary and the vaginal wall. If the pessary descends to the introitus or is expelled, a larger size of the same pessary or a different type of pessary should be tried. If the patient is uncomfortable once the pessary is inserted, it is likely too large and should be replaced with a smaller size. If the pessary remains in place during the Valsalva in the supine position, the test should be repeated after the patient assumes an upright position. Optimally, the patient should be able to ambulate normally and be able to perform a Valsalva in the upright position. Once it is evident that the pessary will remain in place,

patients should be asked to void to ensure that the urethra is not obstructed.

Patients with vaginal atrophy should be given a brief course (2–4 weeks) of local estrogens either prior to fitting or immediately after. This may minimize the side effects of vaginal abrasions and erosions. Instructions concerning pessary care should be given to the patient and a follow-up appointment scheduled.

7.5 FITTING INSTRUCTIONS FOR SPECIFIC PESSARIES

7.5.1 Ring and Ring with Support: Insertion
The ring pessary with or without support is designed to fold along the axis of a straight line drawn between the indentations on the ring and the larger perforations in the ring with support (see Chapter 5, Figure 5.4).

Step 1: With both hands gloved, the pessary is held by the thumb and index finger of the dominant hand in the folded position with the arc facing up (Figure 7.1).

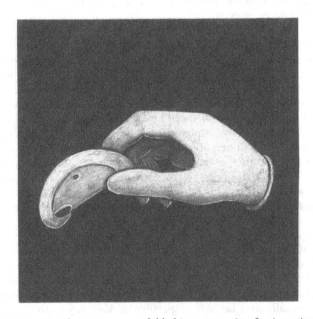

FIGURE 7.1. The ring pessary folded in preparation for insertion.

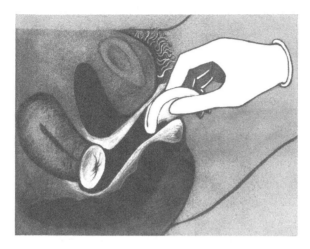

FIGURE 7.2. The ring pessary is rotated into the vagina along the posterior wall.

Step 2: The labia minora are separated at the posterior introitus to reveal the vaginal canal. The pessary is introduced into the vagina parallel to the floor and rotated backward along the posterior vaginal wall (Figure 7.2).

Step 3: As the pessary is advanced into the vagina, the thumb and index finger of the nondominant hand are used to keep the pessary folded to avoid patient discomfort (Figure 7.3). Eventually the pessary is released and advanced into place with the index finger (Figure 7.4).

Step 4: Once the pessary has been introduced into the vagina, its position should be checked. The index finger of the dominant hand is directed into the posterior vaginal fornix, to ensure that the cervix is resting above the pessary (Figure 7.5). It may be necessary to push the pessary beneath the cervix. If difficulty is encountered seating the pessary in the posterior vaginal fornix, it may help to elevate the outer edge of the pessary behind the symphysis pubis, thereby rotating the leading edge of the pessary posteriorly.

Step 5: When the ring pessary is properly placed, the cervix will be in the middle of the ring, supported by the supportive diaphragm when the ring with support is used. The ring can be rotated 90 degrees to orient the folding axis at right angles

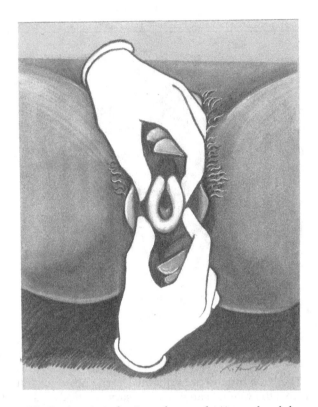

FIGURE 7.3. During introduction, the nondominant hand keeps the pessary folded.

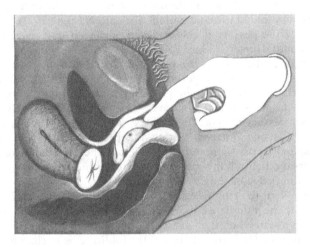

FIGURE 7.4. Ring pessary is advanced into place.

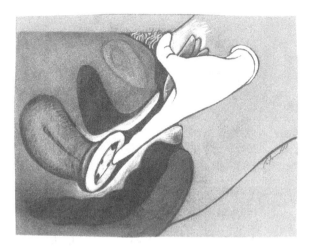

FIGURE 7.5. The proper position and fit of the ring pessary is checked.

to the vaginal canal, though this maneuver has never been shown by experience or research to be necessary. This orientation will make pessary removal by the patient more difficult.

Step 6: The fit of the pessary should be tested. It should be possible to slide the pessary up and down along the vaginal sidewall and to insert a finger between the vaginal sidewall and the pessary. When the labia are separated, a well-supported pessary is not usually visible. When the ring pessary is properly placed it lies along the vaginal axis. It is not usual for it to sit behind the symphysis pubis. During Valsalva testing, the pessary may descend but should return to its proper position when these efforts are stopped. If the pessary descends to the introitus with Valsalva, a larger size should be tried. Routine pessary testing as described previously (section 7.4) should be conducted before discharging the patient.

7.5.2 Ring and Ring with Support: Removal

Step 1: If the pessary has been rotated after insertion, the large perforation in the support diaphragm should be hooked with the index finger (Figure 7.6) and rotated to the midline to line up the folding axis of the pessary with the vaginal canal.

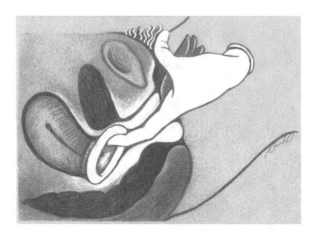

FIGURE 7.6. Ring pessary is hooked with index finger.

Step 2: The index fingers of both hands are inserted into the vagina to hook the leading edge of the ring pessary from above and below. With these fingers, traction is applied to bring the pessary down to the introitus. A push by the patient may help move the pessary down to a point where it can be grasped.

Step 3: Once the pessary has been brought to the introitus it can be grasped with the thumb and index finger of the dominant hand. The nondominant hand is held over the introitus so that its thumb and index finger can be used to fold the ring pessary as it is pulled through the introitus, thus facilitating pessary removal without discomfort (Figure 7.7). Once the pessary is removed it is washed in tap water and dried with a paper towel.

The vaginal walls are inspected using a speculum to look for evidence of abrasions or erosions caused by the pessary. If none are found and the pessary is intact and flexing normally, it is reinserted.

7.5.3 Gellhorn Pessary: Insertion

Step 1: With both hands gloved, the knob of the Gellhorn pessary is held with the thumb and index finger of the dominant hand

(Figure 7.8). With the fingers of the nondominant hand the labia minora are separated and the posterior introitus is depressed. The Gellhorn pessary is oriented transversely to the introitus and at a slightly oblique angle (Figure 7.9).

Step 2: The base of the pessary is introduced over the posterior introitus, and once the leading edge has entered the vagina the pessary should be directed with some pressure along the posterior wall of the vagina until it has passed beneath the inferior pubic rami (Figure 7.10).

Step 3: To finish seating the pessary, the index finger is used to push the knob along the axis of the vagina. When properly seated the base of the Gellhorn pessary will be oriented at right angles to the vaginal canal and the column and knob

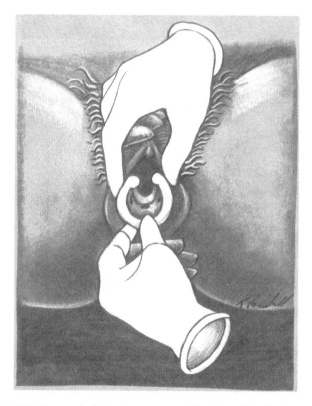

FIGURE 7.7. Removal of the ring pessary is facilitated by flexing it as it slides through the introitus.

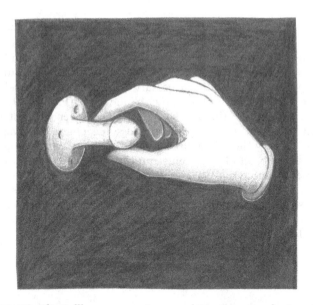

FIGURE 7.8. The Gellhorn pessary is grasped in preparation for insertion.

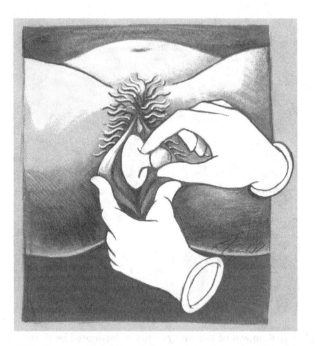

FIGURE 7.9. Fingers of the nondominant hand separate the labia and depress the posterior introitus as the Gellhorn is inserted.

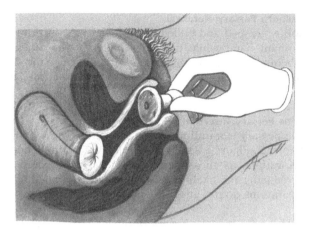

FIGURE 7.10. The Gellhorn pessary slides along the posterior vaginal wall during insertion.

will lie along the vaginal canal with the knob visible at the introitus if the labia are separated (Figure 7.11).

With a Valsalva maneuver the Gellhorn usually does not descend because of the suction effect of its base. The knob may move slightly but should not project out of the introitus. If the Gellhorn is providing good support but the knob is projecting out of the vagina, a model of the same size with a shorter column should be substituted.

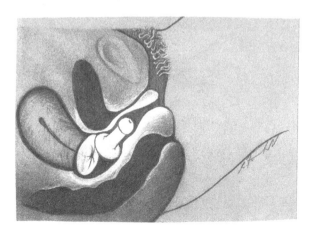

FIGURE 7.11. The Gellhorn pessary properly positioned in the vagina.

7.5.4 Gellhorn Pessary: Removal

The knob is grasped and pulled down toward the introitus with the dominant hand while the index finger of the other hand sweeps behind the base to release any suction. Once the suction is released the pessary is brought out through the introitus by reversing the steps used for insertion.

7.5.5 Cube Pessary: Insertion

The cube pessary is a uniform square with six concave surfaces (see Chapter 5, Figure 5.8). It is preferable to use the model that has perforations as these permit some vaginal secretions to escape, reducing the likelihood of odor and copious discharge. The perforations do not affect the performance of the pessary.

Step 1: The cube pessary is very difficult to reduce in size for insertion. We usually use two hands to attempt to "scrunch" this pessary (Figure 7.12). Once this is achieved, the pessary is held in one hand while the fingers of the other separate the labia and apply downward traction on the posterior vaginal fornix.

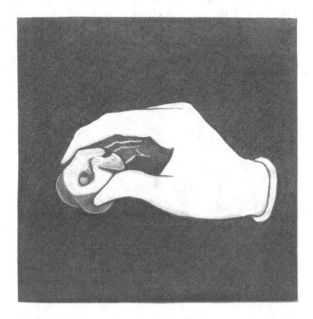

FIGURE 7.12. The cube pessary "scrunched" in preparation for insertion.

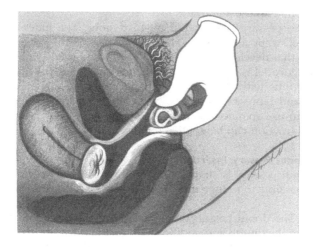

FIGURE 7.13. Insertion of the cube pessary.

Step 2: The pessary is inserted directly into the vagina as far as possible before it is released (Figure 7.13). Once released the index finger is used to alternately push the top and bottom of the pessary to advance it to the top of the vagina. When properly placed the cube comes to rest at the vaginal apex against either the vaginal vault or the cervix (Figure 7.14).

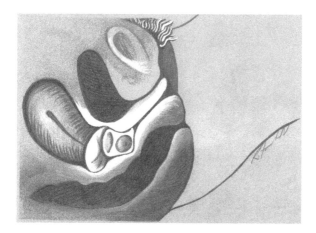

FIGURE 7.14. The cube pessary properly positioned in the vagina.

7.5.6 Cube Pessary: Removal

The cube pessary is very difficult to remove. The index finger must be swept along the sides of the pessary to release the suction that develops between the pessary and the vaginal side-wall (Figure 7.15). The pessary is then grasped and pulled out of the introitus with the dominant hand while the fingers of the other hand depress the posterior vaginal introitus. It is often necessary to use sponge forceps to grasp the cube pessary so that enough traction can be applied for removal.

7.5.7 Donut Pessary: Insertion

The donut pessary is shaped like the inner tube of a tire and it is not possible to reduce the size of this pessary for insertion.

Step 1: The donut pessary is grasped with the dominant hand using the thumb and middle finger on the sides and the index finger in the hole in the middle to direct the pessary (Figure 7.16).

Step 2: The fingers of the other hand are used to separate the labia and to depress the posterior introitus of the vagina. The pessary is inserted directly into the vagina and with the index finger pushed up as high as it will go (Figure 7.17). The donut pessary sits along the vaginal axis with the upper end in contact with either the cervix or the vaginal apex (Figure 7.18).

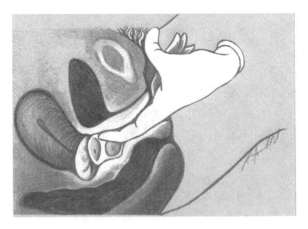

Figure 7.15. Finger inserted to break suction with the vaginal wall.

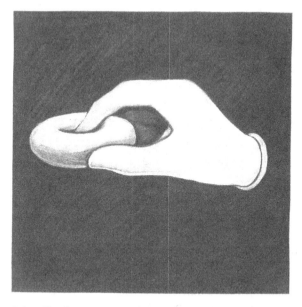

FIGURE 7.16. The donut pessary is grasped in preparation for insertion.

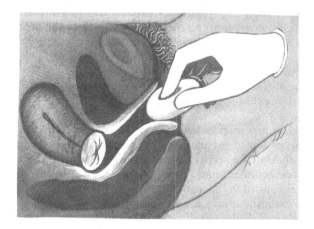

FIGURE 7.17. Insertion of the donut pessary.

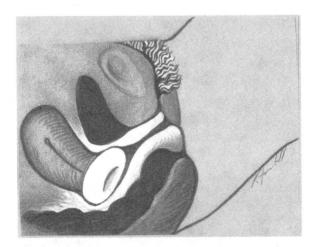

FIGURE 7.18. The donut pessary properly placed in the vagina.

7.5.8 Donut Pessary: Removal

The donut pessary may be difficult to remove because its rounded surfaces making grasping this pessary difficult. If the index finger can be inserted into the hole in the middle of the pessary, it can usually be pulled out. If this is not possible, it may be necessary to visualize the pessary with a speculum and to grasp it with a single tooth tenaculum. As the pessary is pulled out, the posterior introitus should be depressed.

7.5.9 Lever Pessaries: Insertion

Lever pessaries should restricted to the indication of a retroverted uterus that is symptomatic.

Step 1: The first step is to antevert the uterus. If the uterus is incarcerated in pregnancy, this may have to be done under anesthesia. The uterus is held in the anteverted position with the nondominant hand either abdominally or by pressing the cervix toward the sacrum. Alternately, the knee chest position may keep the uterus anteverted.

Step 2: Due to the longitudinal shape of this pessary, size should be determined by measuring the length of the vagina from the posterior fornix to the symphysis pubis. The lever pessary is folded along its longitudinal axis and held with the dominant hand by the index finger and thumb. If the nondominant hand is free, it can be used to separate the labia.

Step 3: The pessary is inserted by directing the leading edge with the index finger of the nondominant hand along the posterior vaginal wall to a position behind the cervix and then elevating the anterior arch behind the symphysis.

Step 4: The uterus should be held in anteversion with the cervix directed posteriorly. The anterior arch should sit comfortably behind the symphysis but not obstruct the urethra. With a Valsalva, the anterior bar should not pass the introitus. Since the risk of compression of the urethra by the anterior bar, especially with the Smith pessary, is considerable, a trial of voiding is absolutely mandatory before the patient leaves the clinic.

7.5.10 Lever Pessaries: Removal

The anterior bar is grasped with one or both index fingers and brought down to the introitus. The pessary is then folded. The nondominant hand is used to separate the labia and the pessary is withdrawn with the dominant hand.

7.6 SUMMARY AND REVIEW OF KEY POINTS

This chapter covered the general procedures used to fit a pessary and the steps used to insert and remove specific commonly used pessaries.

KEY POINTS

1. Pessary fitting is a trial-and-error process that requires the availability of a selection of pessaries.
2. Vaginal atrophy should be treated aggressively with local estrogen replacement to minimize vaginal abrasions.
3. Dry gloves should always be used to minimize loss of pessary control that can result in patient discomfort.
4. Patient comfort and ability to void should be confirmed before discharging a patient after a new pessary fitting.
5. The ring pessary is the only pessary that can be reduced in size for insertion.
6. Removal of the cube and donut pessaries is often difficult and may require the use of an instrument.
7. Lever pessaries should be restricted to cases of symptomatic uterine retroversion.

Chapter 8

Fitting and Care of Continence Pessaries

Baharak Amir-Khalkhali and Scott A. Farrell

8.1 OUTLINE

This chapter discusses the fitting and management of commonly used continence pessaries. The following issues are addressed:

1. General principles of fitting a pessary to treat urinary incontinence
2. The fitting and care of the following specific pessaries:
   a. Incontinence ring pessary
   b. Ring pessary with knob
   c. Incontinence dish
   d. Uresta pessary

8.2 INTRODUCTION

Recent research evidence has demonstrated that pessaries can be used effectively to restore urinary continence (Chapter 3). The continence pessaries that have been studied and are most frequently used include the incontinence ring, the ring pessary with knob, the incontinence dish, and the Uresta pessary. This chapter provides a detailed description of continence pessary fitting, insertion, and removal.

8.3 GENERAL PRINCIPLES OF CONTINENCE PESSARY FITTING

The primary function of a continence pessary is to provide mechanical support to the urethra during activities that increase bladder pressure and threaten to overwhelm the urethral sphincter mechanism. Women with stress urinary incontinence span a much wider age range than those with pelvic prolapse. Younger women are more likely to be sexually active and to experience incontinence intermittently during specific activities. For these reasons, it is very important that a continence pessary design facilitates pessary insertion and removal and minimizes the risk of pessary misplacement.

Patients should be informed about the range of treatment options available for stress incontinence. The continence pessary should be demonstrated to them. They should be given a brief overview of the implications of using a pessary. Pelvic exam should be comprehensive (Chapter 4) and in particular should seek to confirm urethral hypermobility and to assess the extent of pelvic prolapse. As with prolapse pessaries, the length and width of the vagina will determine the size of continence pessary. The patient should be fitted in the lithotomy position. Selection of a pessary is discussed in Chapter 6. After fitting, the effectiveness should be tested first in the supine and then in the standing position. The patient should void to ensure the urethra is not obstructed.

The patient is encouraged to use the pessary for a 2-week trial period, after which she should return for review. If she is satisfied with the effectiveness of the continence pessary, she can be taught to insert and remove the pessary. Patients who are able to manage their pessary independently can be seen on an annual basis for a speculum examination to rule out abrasions in the vaginal canal. For those who are not managing their pessary, follow-up visits should occur at 3- to 6-month intervals.

8.4 INCONTINENCE RING PESSARY: INSERTION

The incontinence ring is composed of a narrow silicone ring enclosing a metal spring to which a knob is affixed (see Chapter 6, Figure 6.1). This pessary is easily compressed at its midpoint for insertion into the vagina.

Step 1: A vaginal exam is performed to assess the vaginal length and caliber. The pessary size is chosen primarily on the basis of vaginal length because it is critically important that the knob sit approximately 1.5 to 2 cm proximal to the urethral meatus. The pessary is introduced by compressing the midpoint of the ring to make it assume an oval shape (Figure 8.1).

Step 2: The end of the pessary opposite to the knob is introduced at a slight angle (approximately 20 degrees above the horizontal) through the posterior vaginal introitus (Figure 8.2) and directed with the index finger of the nondominant hand into the posterior cul-de-sac (Figure 8.3). The knob is pushed farther into the vagina to seat the pessary.

Step 3: The cranial end of the ring should be seated behind the cervix (Figure 3.2). If it rides up over the anterior cervix, the

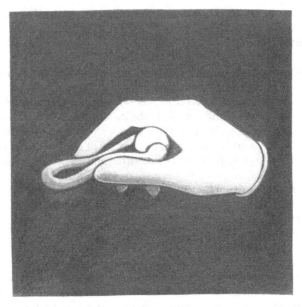

FIGURE 8.1. The incontinence ring is grasped at its midpoint for compression and insertion.

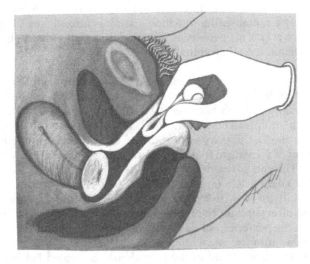

FIGURE 8.2. Ring pessary is inserted along the posterior vagina wall.

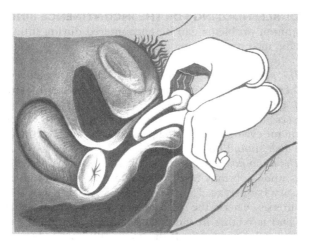

FIGURE 8.3. The ring pessary is directed by the index finger of one hand into the posterior vaginal fornix.

knob will be directed inferiorly away from the urethra where it will be ineffective.

Step 4: Once the pessary is placed, its position should be checked by separation of the labia and inspection of the vaginal introitus. The knob of the pessary is normally not visible when the labia minor are spread with examining fingers. If the knob is visible below the urethral meatus, the pessary is either misplaced or too large. The pessary position should be checked and corrected or a smaller pessary inserted. When properly fitted, the knob can be palpated sitting approximately 1.5 to 2 cm behind the urethral meatus.

Step 5: The effectiveness of the pessary should be tested with the patient first in the supine and then in the standing positions, preferably with a full bladder. The patient should void to ensure that the pessary does not obstruct the urethra. Each patient should receive a set of guidelines for pessary care and follow-up.

8.5 INCONTINENCE RING: REMOVAL

The incontinence ring can be easily hooked with the index finger and pulled down to the introitus where the knob can be grasped and the pessary removed. Because this pessary is very flexible, it does not require any manipulation during removal.

8.6 TROUBLESHOOTING FOR THE INCONTINENCE RING

Two common problems can be encountered during fitting and care of the incontinence ring pessary:

1. *The pessary is pushed out with a Valsalva maneuver.* The incontinence ring is most effective in the absence of any significant pelvic organ prolapse. If it falls out with Valsalva maneuvers, a heavier ring is probably required to support a concomitant cystocele. The ring pessary with knob or the incontinence dish should be substituted.

2. *The knob does not sit under the urethra.* In a patient with a uterus, the knob may be displaced because the cranial end of the pessary is misplaced in the anterior vaginal fornix, in front of the uterus. Check the pessary position to ensure that the cranial end is resting in the posterior fornix behind the cervix (see Chapter 3, Figure 3.2). If the knob still projects beyond the urethral meatus despite proper positioning, substitute a smaller size incontinence ring.

8.7 INCONTINENCE DISH

The incontinence dish pessary is bowl shaped with a central opening and a knob attached (see Chapter 6, Figure 6.3). This pessary is flexible enough to be folded in a fashion similar to the incontinence ring pessary and therefore can be inserted and removed using the technique described for the incontinence ring.

8.8 RING PESSARY WITH KNOB: INSERTION

The ring pessary with knob is a modification of the standard ring pessary by the addition of a knob on one side of the pessary (see Chapter 6, Figure 6.2). Because it must be folded for insertion, and rotated once inserted, it is more difficult to manage.

Step 1: As with the incontinence ring, the vaginal length and caliber are first determined by vaginal exam. The smallest sizes of this pessary (from 0 to 2) are difficult to fold, and direct insertion without folding is usually well tolerated by patients. Using the fingers of one hand to separate the labia and depress the posterior vaginal introitus, the smaller pessaries are held by the knob and inserted along the posterior wall of the vagina. As with the incontinence ring, the knob is pushed up to seat the pessary.

Step 2: The larger sizes of this pessary are folded so that the convex curve faces up with knob on the right side of the folded pessary (Figure 8.4). The thumb and index finger of the nondominant hand are used to keep the pessary folded as it passes through the introitus (Figure 8.5).

Step 3: Because the knob is fixed to the side of the pessary at 90 degrees to its folding axis, once the pessary has been inserted the knob will be oriented at right angles to the vaginal axis and must be rotated anteriorly to sit underneath the urethra (Figure 8.6). After rotation it should be located approximately 1.5 to 2 cm cranial to the urethral meatus as with the incontinence ring (Figure 8.7). Since rotation of the knob from the side to the front is sometimes difficult and uncomfortable for the patient, we use a maneuver that combines the insertion and rotations steps. This is best accomplished with the knob on the right side. As the pessary passes into the vagina the controlling hand releases the ring and rotates the pessary clockwise at the same time so that the knob comes to rest below the urethra. When properly placed, the knob of the pessary should rest in the midline approximately 1.5 to 2 cm proximal to the urethral meatus.

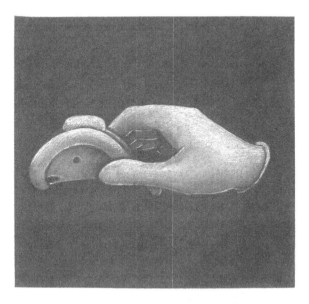

FIGURE 8.4. The ring with support and knob folded for insertion.

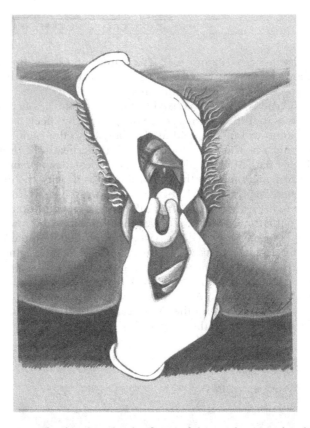

FIGURE 8.5. The thumb and index finger of the nondominant hand keep the pessary folded as it is inserted.

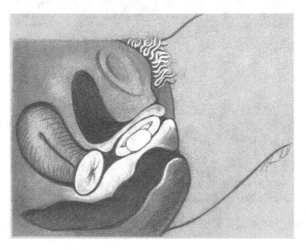

FIGURE 8.6. Orientation of the knob of the ring with knob pessary after insertion.

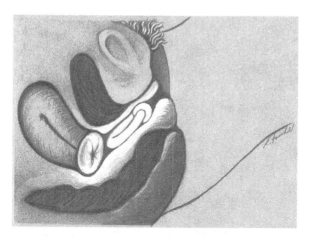

FIGURE 8.7. The ring with support and knob properly placed in the vagina.

8.9 RING PESSARY WITH KNOB: REMOVAL

For removal, the knob must be rotated to the side of the vagina. The pessary is grasped with the index fingers of both hands and pulled down to the introitus. It is then grasped with the thumb and index finger of one hand while the other hand is used to fold the pessary as it is withdrawn. As with the incontinence ring, effectiveness and voiding should be tested before the patient leaves the clinical area. Troubleshooting for this pessary is similar to that for a standard ring pessary.

8.10 URESTA PESSARY: INSERTION

The Uresta pessary is bell-shaped and equipped with a handle at the base of the bell for easy control (see Chapter 6, Figure 6.5). The tapered end of the pessary allows for direct insertion into the vagina like a tampon, a process that is intuitive for women.

Step 1: Vaginal caliber is more critical than vaginal length in the fitting of the Uresta pessary. In most women, it is reasonable to start with a medium sized (No. 4) pessary. A water-soluble lubricant is placed on the tip of the pessary. The pessary handle is grasped with the thumb and index finger of the dominant hand while the fingers of the other hand separate the labia (Figure 8.8).

Step 2: The pessary is directed straight into the vagina with slight pressure on the posterior introitus to help ease it under the symphysis pubis (Figure 8.9). Once it is inserted to the point

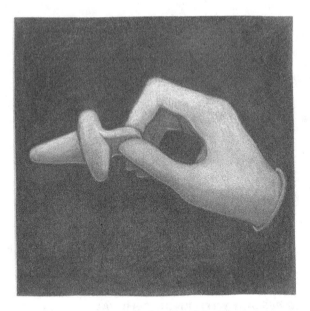

FIGURE 8.8. Grasping the handle of the Uresta pessary.

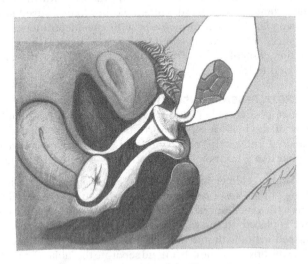

FIGURE 8.9. Insertion of the Uresta pessary.

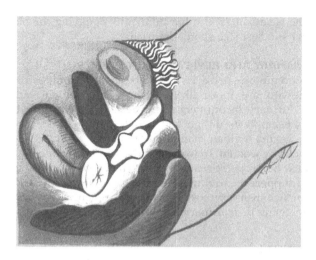

FIGURE 8.10. The Uresta pessary properly positioned in the vagina.

where the handle must be released, it is seated by gently pushing the handle further into the vagina. This pessary does not require manipulation inside the vagina, as it automatically assumes the correct position. When properly fitted a woman should not be aware of the pessary and should be able to empty her bladder without obstruction (Figure 8.10).

8.11 URESTA PESSARY: REMOVAL
Grasping the handle and exerting outward traction while gently bearing down into the pelvis effects pessary removal.

8.12 TROUBLESHOOTING FOR THE URESTA PESSARY
1. *The pessary falls out or is pushed out with straining.* If the Uresta pessary falls out the next larger size should be inserted.

2. *The pessary does not stop leaking.* In most cases where the leaking does not stop when the pessary is inserted, it may be assumed that the pessary is not large enough to provide adequate support to the urethra. A larger size should be tried.

3. *The pessary is uncomfortable.* The pessary may be uncomfortable for one of two reasons: it is too small and is falling down to the introitus or it is too large. In the first case, it usually does not stop the leaking and should be replaced with a larger size. In the second case the pessary is too large. If too large a pessary is

used, the wearer may also have difficulty emptying the bladder. The next smallest size should be tried.

8.13 SUMMARY AND REVIEW OF KEY POINTS

Urinary continence pessaries should be easy to handle as younger women who are more likely to have intermittent, activity-specific, urinary incontinence will be using them. The Uresta pessary, because its design and handle permit direct insertion into the vagina without manipulation, is most likely to be properly placed by women. In women with a uterus, the incontinence ring must be properly seated behind the cervix in order for the knob to support the urethra. The ring pessary with knob and the incontinence dish are most effective in women with a cystocele accompanying their urinary incontinence.

KEY POINTS
1. Larger numbers of younger women with activity-specific bladder leaking will be using continence pessaries. Convenience and ease of use will be more important in this group when compared to women using pessaries for prolapse.
2. The ideal placement of the knob of the continence pessaries is at the midurethra.
3. Annual follow-up is appropriate for asymptomatic women who manage their incontinence ring or Uresta pessary themselves.
4. In order for the knob to support the urethra, the incontinence ring must be properly seated behind the cervix.
5. Uresta's direct insertion and removal, facilitated by its handle, make it the simplest and most intuitive continence pessary.

Chapter 9
Patient Education Regarding Pessary Care

Karen D. Farrell, Linda E. Irving, Jane E. Twohig, and Joan M. Foren

9.1 OUTLINE
This chapter addresses the educational aspects of pessary care. The following issues are discussed:

1. A schedule for pessary follow-up
2. Patient instructions concerning general pessary care
3. Patient instructions concerning pessary insertion and removal
4. A trouble-shooting guide and solutions to common pessary problems
5. Answers to frequently asked questions about pessaries

9.2 INTRODUCTION
Years of experience in a urogynecology clinic lead us to believe that successful pessary use is predicated upon patient education undertaken with women by healthcare professionals after pessary fitting. This education empowers women to use and care for pessaries in a knowledgeable way, increases the likelihood of successful long-term use, and enables women to be active partners in the healthcare relationship. This chapter outlines the educational information that we consider helpful for healthcare professionals to provide to women who have been fitted with a pessary for prolapse or urinary incontinence. The information is designed to enhance women's understanding of what a pessary is, what it will do for them, how to care for it, the types of problems they might encounter with a pessary, and what to do about those problems. A trouble-shooting guide and questions frequently asked by patients regarding pessaries are included in this chapter.

9.3 GUIDELINES FOR WOMEN AT TIME OF INITIAL PESSARY FITTING

9.3.1 Schedule of Pessary Visits

Women are advised that following their initial visit for fitting, pessary checks at 2 weeks, 3 months, 6 months, and 1 year are required for optimal pessary follow-up and care. After 1 year of successful, uneventful pessary use if women are inserting, removing, and caring for the pessary themselves and are not experiencing any problems, they are asked to return for pessary checks annually. If women are not inserting and removing the pessary themselves, they are asked to return for follow-up at 3-month intervals. Women are advised that if they experience any adverse events between follow-up visits (e.g., pessary falls out; bleeding; malodorous discharge; pain; difficulty with voiding or bowel movements), they are to arrange an earlier appointment with a healthcare professional either at the gynecology clinic or with their family physician.

9.3.2 Pessary Care

Patients are given a brief, simple, illustrated explanation of where pessaries are placed in their bodies (in the vagina) and how pessaries work. Patients are given an opportunity to view a pessary. Patients are advised that pessaries are made from either medical-grade silicone or rubber (not latex) and that allergic reaction to them or infection from them is uncommon.

Women are told that the material pessaries are made of is not odor absorbing. However, normal moisture in the vagina will collect on a pessary and over a period of time can cause odor or discharge. This discharge may have a natural vaginal odor, which is not out of the ordinary, and patients should not be alarmed. To prevent it, patients are advised to remove the pessary at least once weekly, wash it with water and soap then soak it in a mixture of vinegar and water (half and half), dry it well, and leave it in a container overnight. If they don't wish to remove the pessary themselves, they have the option of douching one or two times per week with warm water to wash the discharge out. If the problem persists, there are preparations that may be prescribed by a physician to address the vaginal discharge and odor (e.g., Trimosan vaginal gel (Milex, Chicago, Illinois, USA), Vagifem (Novo Nordisk, Novo Allé, Denmark), or the Estring (Pfizer, New York, New York, USA)). Women should be reassured that the Vagifem and Estring products are local estrogen replacement products that are not absorbed systemically.

9.3.3 Pessary Fit

Before initial fitting, women are asked if they have ever used a tampon or a diaphragm. This question helps to assess the comfort level of patients with the notion of touching their own bodies and using a vaginal device like a pessary. Women who have used and are comfortable with tampons or diaphragms are often more at ease with the process of inserting and removing a vaginal pessary than those who have not.

After initial fitting, patients are advised to use the pessary for 2 weeks and to do their normal activities. If they experienced urine leakage before the initial pessary fitting, they are advised to "test" their pessary by doing the activities that precipitated urine loss to see if they still have urine leakage with the pessary in place. During the 2 weeks, if patients have any urine leakage with the pessary in place or if the pessary descends, it may be necessary to try another size or type of pessary. It may take trial and error to determine the correct pessary size/type and to see if this treatment option works well for them. Patients are advised that pessaries are only one treatment option for urinary incontinence or prolapse. If pessaries do not work for them or they don't wish to use this treatment option, then other options like surgery should be discussed with a physician.

Patients are advised that if pessaries are fitted properly, they should not feel them inside their body. However, it is possible for pessaries to dislodge or fall out with tremendous straining (e.g., during bowel movements, vigorous exercise, or activity involving lifting). Patients are advised that at first they should check the toilet each time before flushing, especially after bowel movements, to be sure that the pessary has not fallen out. If they feel the pessary coming down, they can put their hands over the vaginal opening to keep the pessary from dropping into the toilet. Patients who have chronic constipation and wish to use a pessary are advised to try to correct the constipation problem through diet (increase fiber and fluids) and lifestyle changes (increase physical activity).

If the pessary is dislodged by straining and descends, it will not work as well as it should. So if patients notice that the pessary has descended, feels different, or is not working as well, they are advised to try to adjust the position of the pessary to see if it fixes the problem. The pessary may be safely pushed back into place by inserting a finger into the vagina and gently pushing the pessary upward. If the problem is not fixed, then a change in the style or size of pessary may be needed and the patient is advised to see their healthcare professional. Patients are shown how to remove the pessary in case it becomes uncomfortable or they decide not to use it for any reason. If the pessary interferes with bowel movements or voiding, it should be removed.

9.3.4 Pessary Insertion and Removal

If patients are willing to care for their pessary themselves, they are shown how to insert and remove it. Additionally, patients may be given the package insert from their pessary and an incontinence pessary care handbook for their particular type of pessary. The handbook contains educational information and written and pictorial instructions about how to insert and remove the pessary. Like removing a tampon, patients are told to stand and put a foot up on the closed lid of the toilet in their bathroom to insert or remove their pessary. Alternatively, they can sit leaning forward on the edge of the toilet lid or on a chair to insert or remove the pessary. For women who find these positions difficult, it is recommended they lie on their bed propped up with pillows so that their head and shoulders are raised up. This position makes it easier to reach the vagina and to insert or remove the pessary. It is recommended that they place a clean towel beneath them to protect the bed. The key thing to convey to patients is not to panic if they have difficulty removing the pessary. No harm will come to them if they cannot remove it. They should be counseled that if they are experiencing discomfort or pain, they should try to reposition the pessary by pushing gently with their fingers and to see a healthcare professional.

Potential problems with pessaries and the solutions to those problems are discussed with patients (see Trouble-Shooting Guide, section 9.5). Patients are advised that their pessary may not be "sexual intercourse friendly." Some patients and their partners are not bothered by the presence of a pessary and are able to comfortably leave the pessary in the vagina during sexual intercourse. Other patients and their partners prefer to remove the pessary for sexual activity. If left in during sexual intercourse, douching should be done sometime afterward.

Patients are cautioned that continence pessaries may not make their incontinence problem 100% better. The urine leakage may be stopped entirely or it may only be reduced to a more manageable level. This reduction may be acceptable, especially if other options such as surgery are contraindicated. Patients are advised to take the package insert and pessary care booklet with them if they find it necessary to visit a healthcare professional for pessary care.

9.4 FIRST FOLLOW-UP VISIT

At the time of the first follow-up visit at 2 weeks, patients are asked how they managed with their pessary and if they experienced any problems (e.g., discharge, odor, difficulty inserting or removing). Patients are given an opportunity to ask questions, and educational information about pessaries and pessary care is reviewed. If patients have not been caring for their pessary themselves but express an interest in doing so, they are instructed in the insertion, removal, and care of it. After removal of the pessary, a speculum examination is conducted by a healthcare professional to inspect the health of the vagina and to look for abrasions or erosions. If no problems are found, the pessary is reinserted. The removal and reinsertion may be done by the patient or healthcare professional, depending on patient preference. If done by the patient, the pessary positioning is checked by the healthcare professional. Patients are advised to call with any questions or for further clarification or reinforcement of the pessary teaching.

9.5 TROUBLE-SHOOTING GUIDE: POTENTIAL PROBLEMS AND THEIR SOLUTIONS

9.5.1 Difficulty Removing Pessary

Some patients find it difficult to remove their pessaries. For these patients the following hint has proved to be helpful. It is suggested they tie a piece of twill tape, dental floss, fishing line, or I.V. tubing around the pessary to help them pull it out. Women are advised to change the string/tape when they clean their pessary weekly. The I.V. tubing may be washed thoroughly and reused.

9.5.2 Pessary Falls Out

Patients are advised that if their pessary falls out to wash it off with water and soap, dry it thoroughly, wrap it up, and bring it with them to the clinic. A change in the size or type of pessary may be required.

9.5.3 Discomfort Using Pessary

Discomfort may arise if the pessary shifts out of its correct position in the vagina. If willing to do so, patients may reposition the pessary by inserting a finger into the vagina and pushing the pessary back into place. Alternatively, they may try removing the pessary and reinserting it in the correct position. If unwilling to do this adjustment themselves, they may return to the clinic. A change in the size or type of pessary may be needed to find a more comfortable fit.

9.5.4 Pelvic Pain

Patients are advised to remove the pessary and notify the clinic if they experience pain. If they are unable to remove the pessary, they are told to come to the clinic or go to their family doctor or local emergency room for removal. A change in pessary size or type may be needed.

9.5.5 Vaginal Discharge or Odor

Vaginal discharge and odor most often occur in women who are not inserting and removing their pessaries themselves. It is not unusual for the discharge to be intermittent, not constant. Patients are advised that discharge and odor is a possibility and an explanation of why it occurs is given (see Pessary Care, section 9.3.2). Patients are advised to douche with warm water mixed with a small amount of vinegar. If vaginal odor and discharge persist, then Trimosan vaginal gel may be prescribed by a physician.

In the uncommon instance of a more severe discharge that is greenish in color and extremely foul-smelling or one that is watery and fishy-smelling, patients are told they should see their physician, who may prescribe antibiotics. Although pessaries do not cause yeast infections, patients may experience one and if they have a white, curdy discharge, they are advised to see their doctor.

9.5.6 Vaginal Bleeding

Vaginal bleeding may be caused by a friction rub (abrasion) from the pessary. It can produce discharge and minimal amounts of bleeding (i.e., streaks of blood). Natural bacteria in the vagina may enter the site of an abrasion and cause an odor. Patients are told this and they are advised not to panic, for in the majority of cases bleeding is from a superficial abrasion. They should see their healthcare professional within a reasonable amount of time. Physicians may prescribe Vagifem to thicken the lining of the vagina and decrease the likelihood that abrasions occur. A short holiday from the pessary may be indicated to allow the vagina to heal. If the bleeding is heavier, patients are advised to see their physicians promptly. If there are no abrasions or erosions found to explain the bleeding, patients with a uterus may require an endometrial biopsy.

9.5.7 Leaking from the Bladder

It is possible for the knob of an incontinence pessary to shift out of the correct position in the vagina, resulting in leaking from the bladder. If this happens, patients are advised to check to see if they can feel the knob of the pessary in the middle of their vagina under their urethra. The pessary may need to be removed and reinserted. Or the size of pessary may have to be changed. Women are advised to consult their healthcare professional if the pessary continually moves out of its correct position resulting in urinary leakage.

9.5.8 General Advice to Patients Regarding Pessaries

Patients are advised that they may wear their pessaries during their menses or remove them, if preferred. They may find it possible to wear a tampon with the pessary in place, particularly with the ring, ring with knob, and incontinence ring pessaries. It is unlikely that wearing a tampon would be possible with any of the space-occupying pessaries such as the Gellhorn, donut, cube, or the Uresta pessary. It is recommended that patients take their pessary out after their period is over, wash it thoroughly, and allow it to dry before reinserting.

Patients sometimes complain that their pessary does not sit like it does in the pictures in the pessary care handbook or package insert. Patients should be told that as long as the pessary is not causing them any problems and it is doing what they want it to do (i.e., reducing the prolapse or stopping the urine leakage), then it does not matter how it sits. It may be individual differences in anatomy that result in variations in positioning within the body. The key thing to consider is, "Is it working?" Similarly, patients often express the belief that the pessary should lie transverse when it actually follows the up-and-down position in the vagina. They should be told that they will only feel the edge of the pessary when they insert their fingers into the vagina. It often helps patients' understanding of how the pessary sits in the body to lay the pessary upon one's abdomen to demonstrate its positioning.

Long-term pessary users may experience sudden changes in effectiveness of their pessary and a change in style or size of pessary may be beneficial at that time. However, sudden changes in bladder function may be the result of a urinary tract infection and not the fault of their pessary; therefore, infection must be ruled out first. Patients are advised to see their healthcare professional to check for the presence of a urinary tract infection before seeking changes in their pessary.

9.6 FREQUENTLY ASKED QUESTIONS

9.6.1 Do I Have to Remove My Own Pessary? How Often Must I Take It Out?

If women don't wish to remove their pessaries themselves, they are advised to douche one or two times per week with warm water to wash any discharge out and to return to the clinic for follow-up at 3-month intervals (see section 9.3.1). Women are also advised that if they experience any adverse events (e.g., pessary falls out, bleeding, malodorous discharge, pain, difficulty with voiding or bowel movements) between follow-up visits, they are to arrange an appointment with a healthcare professional at the clinic or see their family physician.

If caring for their pessary themselves, patients are advised to remove the pessary at least once per week, wash it with water and soap and soak it in a mixture of vinegar and water (half and half), dry it well, and leave in a container overnight.

9.6.2 How Does the Pessary Work? Will It Affect My Ability to Pee or Have a Bowel Movement?

Patients are told the pessaries for prolapse (e.g., ring, gellhorn, cube, donut) work by fitting in the vagina and providing support to the pelvic organs that are falling down or falling out. Incontinence pessaries (e.g., incontinence ring) stop urine leakage from the bladder by supporting the bladder neck (urethra) so that it doesn't sag downward and open with increased intraabdominal pressure caused by activities such as coughing, hearty laughing, sneezing, or lifting. If properly fitted, the patient should not feel the pessary inside the body and it should not interfere with voiding or bowel movements. Patients are advised that if the pessary does interfere with bowel movements or voiding, it should be removed. The pessary size may need to be adjusted.

9.6.3 Can I Have Sex with the Pessary In?

Patients are told that it is possible to leave their pessary in during sexual intercourse but that some pessaries are more "sexual intercourse friendly" than others. It is really a matter of trial and error and personal preference. Some patients and their partners are not bothered by the presence of the pessary and are able to comfortably leave the pessary in the vagina during sexual intercourse. Other patients and their partners prefer to remove the pessary for sexual activity. If left in during sexual intercourse, patients are advised to douche afterward.

9.6.4 Does It Go Anywhere Else in My Body? Can I Put It in the Wrong Place?

Patients are told that the vagina is a closed space, that there is nowhere else for the pessary to go, and they need not worry about the pessary "wandering" elsewhere in their body. The pessary may move out of its correct position (e.g., descend or knob may rotate) but it can be readjusted by simply inserting a finger into the vagina and pushing gently upward or rotating the knob back into position.

9.6.5 Will the Pessary Cause Infection?

Patients should be advised that pessaries are made from either medical-grade silicone or rubber (not latex) and that allergic reaction to them or infection from them is uncommon. However, patients should be counseled to come for care if they experience a discharge that is greenish in color and extremely foul-smelling or one that is watery and fishy-smelling. Their physician will conduct a pelvic exam and may prescribe antibiotics. Although pessaries do not cause yeast infections, patients may experience one, and if they have a white, curdy discharge, they should see their doctor for treatment of it.

9.6.6 What Do I Do If the Pessary Falls Out or I Can't Get It Out?

Patients are advised that if their pessary falls out to wash it off with water and soap, dry it thoroughly, wrap it up, and bring it with them to the clinic. A change in the size or type of pessary may be required.

If patients have difficulty removing their pessary, the key thing to convey to them is not to panic. No harm will come to them if they cannot remove it. They can have it removed by their healthcare professional. If they experience discomfort or pain with the pessary, they should first try to relieve the discomfort by repositioning the pessary (push it gently with their fingers) and then see a healthcare professional for removal.

9.6.7 Will a Pessary Hurt? Will I Feel It?

If properly fitted, patients do not feel pessaries inside their bodies. If a pessary hurts or causes discomfort, patients may need to have the size or type of pessary adjusted or changed, so they should see their healthcare professional.

9.6.8 How Often Will I Need a New Pessary?

The pessary manufacturers suggest a pessary, if cared for properly, will last 2 years before it needs to be replaced. Patients are told this and are advised to have regular pessary checks with their healthcare professional so the pessary integrity may be examined.

9.6.9 What Do I Do If My Pessary Is Not Helping My Bladder?

If the pessary was previously working to stop the urine leakage but no longer seems to be doing so, then the patient is advised to check the position of the pessary in the vagina. It may have rotated out of position and the knob may not be supporting the bladder neck as it should (i.e., it may not be sitting in the middle of the vagina). For long-term pessary users, a change in size or type of pessary may be needed. The possibility of a urinary tract infection must also be ruled out so patients should see their healthcare professional.

For some women, pessaries will not work to stop bladder leaking despite adjustments in size or type. However, all size adjustments and combinations of pessary types should be tried before reaching this conclusion. For women for whom surgery is contraindicated but pessaries do not work to stop the urine leakage completely, reducing the urine leakage to a more manageable amount may still be a reasonable solution if the patient is satisfied with this reduction.

9.7 SUMMARY

Pessaries are a valuable tool in the treatment and management of prolapse and urinary incontinence. With proper education and counseling about the use and care of pessaries, women can successfully use this relatively effortless, nonthreatening treatment option to restore their functioning and improve their quality of life.

Glossary

De novo stress incontinence—stress incontinence that happens for the first time after some intervention such as surgery.

Detrusor instability—a urodynamic term for the inability of a person to stop the bladder from contracting and emptying.

Evisceration—when the bowel protrudes through an opening in the vagina or the abdomen.

Fistula—an abnormal connection between two organs, e.g., a hole connecting the bladder to the vagina.

Hormone replacement therapy—the use of estrogen either systematically (pills, patches, gels) or in the vagina (rings, tablets, creams) to treat conditions caused by a lack of estrogen. Vaginal thinning or atrophy is often treated with local estrogen in the vagina.

Hypoestrogenism—usually refers to conditions caused by a lack of estrogen such as a thin vaginal wall.

Hysterectomy—surgical removal of the uterus and cervix.

Intraabdominal pressure—pressure generated inside the abdomen by a cough or the action of lifting, which pushes on the pelvic organs.

Introitus—the opening of the vagina.

Latent stress incontinence—stress incontinence that is not symptomatic until pelvic prolapse is corrected either with a pessary or by surgery.

Life table analysis—a method of accurately determining the likelihood of a particular outcome that takes into account study dropouts and different duration of follow-up.

Pelvic floor exercises—contraction of the muscles that form the support platform at the bottom of the pelvis on which the pelvic organs rest. Most often used to treat stress incontinence.

Pelvic organ prolapse—occurs when the pelvic organs (uterus, bladder, rectum) descend or bulge out from their normal positions in the pelvis; the organ that is prolapsing determines the name given to the prolapse:

Bladder—cystocele or anterior vaginal wall defect.

Rectum—rectocele or posterior vaginal wall defect.

Uterus—uterine prolapse.

Vaginal vault—vaginal vault or apical prolapse.

Pelvic pressure—a symptom of heaviness or loss of normal support that is felt generally in the lower pelvis by women with pelvic prolapse.

Perineal support—the perineum is the muscles and tissues that lie between the vagina and the rectum. This area should not normally bulge out or descend with straining or coughing.

Pessaries—devices made of silicone in a variety of shapes, which are inserted in the vagina to support the pelvic organs.

Pop-Q—a system for quantifying the location and extent of pelvic organ prolapse by means of nine measurements.

Posterior defect—a bulge on the posterior wall of the vagina where the rectum lies.

Proximal urethra—the urethra is the tube at the bottom of the bladder through which urine flows to outside the body. The proximal urethra is the portion closest to where it attaches to the bladder.

Space-occupying pessary—a pessary that because of its shape and size fills the vagina and expands it.

Splint—the act of inserting fingers into the vagina to support the vaginal wall over an organ such as the bladder or rectum.

Stage III/IV—pelvic organ prolapse severity is usually categorized based on the extent that the prolapse is visible to an examiner:

  Stage I—visible with a speculum in the vagina.

  Stage II—visible at the opening of the vagina.

  Stage III—extending out of the vagina.

  Stage IV—complete loss of support (e.g., vaginal turned completely inside out).

Stress incontinence—leaking of urine from the bladder that happens during coughing, sneezing, or activities such as running and is caused by a failure of the urethra to stay closed.

Support pessary—a pessary that lies along the axis of the vagina with one end in the posterior vaginal fornix and the other beneath the pubic symphysis.

Urethral closure pressure—the difference in pressure between the bladder and the urethra. The urethral pressure is normally higher and this keeps the urethra closed.

Urethrovesical junction—the place where the bladder and urethra join.

Urge urinary incontinence—leaking from the bladder that occurs when a woman is unable to prevent her bladder from contracting on the way to the bathroom.

Urinary continence mechanism—the muscles and tissues that together keep the bladder closed to stop urine from leaking.

Urodynamics testing—tests that use small catheters inserted into the bladder to measure pressures and observe bladder function.

Vaginal compartment—the vagina is often described as having compartments:

  Anterior—front wall of the vagina.

  Apical—top of the vagina.

  Posterior—back wall of the vagina.

Voiding dysfunction—the failure of an organ such as the bladder to empty in the normal way.

Index

Page numbers followed by f indicate figures.